I0711805

Table of Contents:

Welcome to the magical world of infant sleep, a realm of sweetness and calm that can pose a challenge for many first-time parents. Are you ready to uncover secrets and effective strategies to help your baby sleep and rediscover the peace of nighttime rest?

"The Happy Nap: Helping Your Baby Sleep Well with Effective Techniques and Theories for Infant Sleep - A Comprehensive Guide to Bedtime" is a valuable resource for parents aiming to provide their newborn with restful and rejuvenating sleep, without sacrificing moments of serenity for themselves. Written with passion and expertise by renowned author in the field of child care, Anna Silvestri, this book offers an extraordinary journey into the world of infant sleep, providing a comprehensive overview of practical strategies and fundamental theories to ensure a happy nap for every little one.

A Comprehensive Guide to Infant Sleep

The first months of a baby's life are a magical and special time, but it can also be an overwhelming and hectic experience for parents. Understanding your little one's sleep needs is crucial for their healthy and harmonious development. In this guide, you will discover how to establish effective evening routines, create a comfortable environment, and provide the right amount of affection and attention to gently lull your baby to sleep.

The Author, an Authorized Voice

Anna Silvestri is a recognized authority in the field of infancy and newborns, and her passion for helping families overcome infant sleep challenges shines through every page of this book. With extensive experience working with children and parents, Anna has dedicated years to researching and developing innovative techniques to address infant sleep difficulties. Her expertise and empathy make her the perfect ally for parents seeking a reliable and competent guide.

A Unique and Personalized Approach

Every child is a unique individual, and this guide recognizes and embraces this truth. With a flexible and personalized approach, you will learn to identify your baby's specific needs and create a tailor-made evening routine for them. Forget about rigid and standardized methods, and embrace a loving and sensitive approach that takes into account the peculiarities and preferences of your little one.

Proven and Effective Strategies

"Infant Sleep" is a treasure trove of proven and effective strategies to help your baby sleep. From the importance of a stable evening routine to secrets for recognizing your baby's sleep signals, to the art of soothing them with gentleness and patience, each chapter is

infused with valuable knowledge that you can apply in your daily life.

Beyond Sleep: The Power of a Happy Nap

Infant sleep is much more than mere rest. This book explores the crucial role of sleep in your child's growth and development. You will discover how a happy nap can positively impact their physical and mental health, cognitive abilities, and emotional growth. Rejuvenating sleep can also benefit you as a parent, improving your overall health and well-being.

Explore and Experiment

"Infant Sleep" invites you to explore and experiment, to follow your instincts as a parent and adapt strategies to fit you and your baby. There is no one-size-fits-all answer, but there is a rewarding journey to discover what works best for you and your little one. Each chapter is enriched with practical exercises and real-life examples to help you apply the acquired

knowledge and develop a unique and special bedtime routine.

A Journey Towards a Happy Nap

Get ready to embark on a journey towards a happy nap with Anna Silvestri. This comprehensive and detailed guide will lead you step by step through a world of love, tenderness, and understanding, providing you with the tools and knowledge needed to gently and successfully put your baby to sleep.

1.1 The Importance of Sleep in the First Year of Life

The first year of a newborn's life is a period of rapid physical and neurological development and change. During these months, sleep plays a crucial role in numerous fundamental processes, influencing the child's growth, development, and overall well-being. One of the main reasons why sleep is so essential for infants relates to physical growth. While the baby sleeps, the body releases growth hormone, crucial for the development of bones and muscles. This explains why infants who sleep adequately often exhibit healthy and robust growth rates.

From a neurological perspective, sleep helps consolidate the new neural connections formed during waking hours. Every new experience, face, sound, or sensation contributes to forming intricate networks in the baby's brain. During sleep, these connections are strengthened, allowing the newborn to process information, store memories, and learn more effectively. Additionally, during sleep, the brain actively works to eliminate toxins accumulated during the day, a process essential for maintaining optimal brain function. In infants, where the brain is in a constant state of growth and development, this "cleaning" process is particularly vital.

Another key aspect of sleep in the first year relates to emotional regulation and the baby's temperament. It has been observed that infants who sleep well tend to be calmer, less irritable, and generally happier. Conversely, sleep deprivation can lead to increased irritability, frustration, and difficulties in social interaction, negatively impacting both the child and the entire family.

The newborn's immune system also derives significant benefits from adequate sleep. Proper sleep enhances the body's natural defenses, making the baby less susceptible to infections and illnesses. In a period when the immune *system is still developing, ensuring that the newborn gets all the rest they need is crucial for their overall health.*

In conclusion, sleep in the first year of life is not merely a restful period. It is a crucial time of growth, development, and consolidation, preparing the newborn to interact with the external world effectively and healthily. Understanding the importance of this phase makes it clear how essential it is to provide infants with optimal conditions for peaceful and restorative sleep. Moving on to point 1.2, it is equally crucial to understand how the sleep cycles of infants differ from those of adults, as this understanding allows us to adjust our expectations and strategies to the specific needs of the little ones. Once the foundations of sleep are clear, it becomes easier to address potential obstacles and ensure an ideal sleep environment.

1.2 Newborn Sleep Cycles: How They Differ from Adults

When we observe a newborn sleeping, we might be tempted to think that their sleep is a continuous, peaceful, and deep state, but in reality, it is quite different from adult sleep. Understanding the specifics of infant sleep is crucial for managing expectations and establishing appropriate routines. Sleep, both for infants and adults, is divided into different phases. However, the proportions of these phases and their duration differ significantly between newborns and adults.

REM vs. Non-REM Sleep: Sleep is primarily divided into two types: Rapid Eye Movement (REM) sleep and Non-REM sleep. In adults, REM sleep represents only a fraction of the total sleep time, but in newborns, about half of their sleep is REM. This type of sleep, also known as "active sleep," is associated with dreams and is a crucial phase for the baby's brain development.

Short Sleep Cycles: While adults go through sleep cycles lasting 90-120 minutes, newborns have much shorter cycles, typically 50-60 minutes. This means that infants go through phases of light and deep sleep more frequently, making them more susceptible to waking up.

Sleep Needs: During the first months of life, a newborn may sleep up to 16-18 hours a day, divided between daytime naps and nighttime periods. This contrasts with the 7-9 hours of recommended sleep for most adults.

Maturation of Circadian Rhythm: At birth, newborns do not have a well-defined circadian rhythm, the natural system that regulates the sleep-wake cycle in response to light and darkness. In the early months, infants may sleep at intervals both during the day and night. Gradually, with the influence of natural light and daily routines, they will begin to develop a more predictable rhythm.

Waking for Feeding: The capacity of a newborn's stomach to hold food is limited, meaning they will wake frequently for feeding, both day and night. These wake-ups are entirely natural and necessary for their rapid growth rate.

These differences in sleep patterns can sometimes surprise and tire new parents, especially when comparing them to adult sleep habits. However, it is vital to remember that these sleep patterns are normal and represent a crucial phase in the infant's development.

As we move on to section 1.3, we will explore the stages of infant sleep development, understanding how they change over the months, and how parents can expect and manage these changes. Understanding this evolution will help parents create an optimal sleep environment and adapt their routines as the newborn grows.

1.3 Understanding the Phases of Neonatal Sleep Development

Sleep is a dynamic and continually evolving process, especially during the first year of life. In this phase, infants go through various transitions in their sleep patterns, reflecting their overall growth and development. Let's examine these phases to gain a clear overview.

Newborn Sleep (0-2 months): During the first weeks of life, newborns sleep many hours a day without a distinction between day and night. Their primary need is to feed, so they wake frequently for feeding. In this phase, the duration of REM sleep is very high, as it is crucial for their brain development.

Infant Sleep (2-4 months): In this phase, a certain predictability in the sleep-wake rhythm begins to emerge. Infants may start sleeping for longer periods at night and taking more consistent naps during the day. However, nighttime awakenings for feeding remain common and necessary.

Stabilization of Circadian Rhythm (4-6 months):
Around 4-6 months, many infants begin to develop a more defined circadian rhythm. This means they are more inclined to sleep at night and stay awake during the day. Some may even start "sleeping through the night," although this is not guaranteed and varies from individual to individual.

Consolidated Daytime Naps (6-9 months):
As infants grow, the need for daytime sleep typically consolidates into 2-3 well-defined naps. These naps are crucial for their well-being and development, providing rest breaks between play and learning sessions.

Approaching the First Birthday (9-12 months):
As they approach their first birthday, many infants reduce the number of daytime naps to 1 or 2. Their total sleep needs may decrease slightly, and most infants of this age sleep longer during the night.

These phases are generalizations, and every child is unique. Some may require more sleep than others, and transitions may occur at slightly different times. However, a basic understanding of sleep phases helps parents have realistic expectations and prepare for changes.

While these transitions may seem natural and linear on paper, in practice, they can present challenges. Adapting to new sleep routines can give rise to common sleep-related issues. If left unaddressed, these issues can have repercussions not only on the child but also on the entire family. We will explore these issues in more detail in section 1.4, providing a clear insight into potential difficulties and solutions to overcome them. Being aware of these challenges in advance can help parents feel more prepared and respond with empathy and understanding to the continually evolving needs of their little one.

1.4 Common Sleep-Related Issues and Their Impact on the Child and Family

Addressing sleep issues in the first months and years of a newborn's life is a reality that nearly every parent must contend with. These problems not only affect the newborn but can also have profound repercussions on the entire family dynamic.

Frequent Awakenings: As mentioned earlier, it is normal for newborns to wake up during the night, especially in the early months, for feeding. However, frequent awakenings may persist even after the child has passed the phase of needing nighttime feeding. This can be stressful for parents and disrupt the sleep of the entire family.

Difficulty Falling Asleep: Some newborns may have difficulty calming down and falling asleep, even when clearly tired. This could be due to various reasons, such as colic, established sleep habits, or environmental sensitivities.

Nap Transitions: As a child grows and their sleep needs change, they might struggle with transitioning from three naps a day to two, and eventually to one. These transitions can lead to periods of overtiredness or inconsistent sleep.

Night Terrors and Nightmares: Although more common in toddlers than in newborns, episodes of intense fear can manifest and be very distressing for parents. Unlike nightmares, during night terrors, children do not fully wake up and often do not remember the event the next morning.

Dependency on Rituals: Some children may become strongly attached to specific sleep rituals, such as being rocked or listening to a particular lullaby. If these rituals become too elaborate, they can make it challenging for the child to fall asleep in other situations.

The impact of these sleep issues extends beyond the child. Sleep deprivation can cause stress, irritability, and exhaustion in parents. This can lead to tension between partners and affect their ability to function effectively during the day, both at home and at work. Additionally, siblings of the newborn may be disturbed by nighttime awakenings, affecting their well-being and making family routine management even more complex.

Understanding these issues and their causes is the first step in addressing them. Every child is an individual, and what works for one family may not be effective for another. However, with the right strategies and a good dose of patience, these issues can be managed or even overcome. That's why this book aims to provide a comprehensive guide for parents.

In section 1.5, we will explore the main objective of this manual and how it can serve as an essential tool to navigate through the complexities of infant sleep, offering solutions, *strategies, and a deep understanding of the needs of their little ones. The guide will be a compass to navigate through these crucial early years of life, ensuring optimal well-being for the newborn and the entire family.*

1.5 Objective of the Book: Providing a Comprehensive Guide for Parents

Parenthood is one of the most rewarding but also one of the most challenging experiences. Every parent aspires to offer the best to their child, ensuring their well-being and happiness. One of the primary challenges that every parent must face, especially in the first months and years of a child's life, is related to sleep. As we have seen in the previous sections, understanding and managing infant sleep are complex and multifaceted aspects.

The goal of this book is to become a trusted companion for parents on this journey. But what are the specific objectives we hope to achieve with this guide?

Education: First and foremost, we aim to educate parents about the dynamics of infant sleep. Understanding the biological processes, rhythms, and developmental stages helps set realistic expectations and respond empathetically to the child's needs.

Personalized Strategies: Every child is unique, and what works for one may not work for another. We want to provide a variety of techniques and advice, allowing parents to choose and customize strategies based on the specific needs of their family.

Emotional Support: Beyond practical advice, this book aims to provide emotional support. Sleep deprivation and challenges related to parenting can lead to feelings of frustration or inadequacy. Recognizing these feelings and offering reassurance is essential.

Long-Term Vision: Although the emphasis is on the early years of life, we want to prepare parents for the future by providing information on how sleep needs change as the child grows.

Community: Lastly, we want to remind parents that they are not alone on this journey. There are many communities, both online and offline, where parents can share experiences, advice, and mutual support.

With these objectives in mind, this book intends to go beyond simple "techniques to put the baby to sleep." It aims to be a comprehensive manual covering all aspects of infant sleep, offering a balanced perspective based on scientific research, real experiences, and a deep understanding of the needs of infants and their families.

As we proceed with the reading, the next chapter will delve into the biological and neurological factors influencing infant sleep. This fundamental understanding will allow us to approach sleep not only as a physical need but as a complex and interconnected process, intrinsically linked to the overall development of the child. Starting from section 2.1, we will begin this exploration, connecting it to everything we have discussed so far and building a solid *foundation on which to base our future strategies and advice.*

2.1 Biological and Neurological Factors

Sleep, seemingly a passive activity, is actually a profoundly complex process influenced by an intricate network of biological and neurological factors. To fully understand the challenges and sleep needs of infants, it is essential to begin with a solid understanding of these aspects.

Circadian Rhythm: Still developing in infants, the circadian rhythm is our internal biological clock that regulates wakefulness and sleep cycles. While in adults this rhythm is well-established (awake during the day, sleepy at night), in infants, it may take time to synchronize with the external day-night cycle. This explains why infants tend to sleep intermittently during both day and night.

Melatonin Production: Melatonin, often referred to as the "sleep hormone," regulates sleep-wake cycles. Its production is influenced by light—it increases in darkness and decreases in light. Infants begin to produce melatonin only a few weeks after birth, which can impact their sleep patterns.

Brain Development and Sleep Stages: The brains of infants go through distinct phases during sleep, including Rapid Eye Movement (REM) sleep and non-REM sleep. REM sleep, associated with dreams, is crucial for brain development and constitutes a significantly higher percentage of total sleep in infants compared to adults.

Neurotransmitters: These chemicals in the brain play an essential role in sleep regulation. For instance, adenosine accumulates in the brain during wakefulness and promotes sleep when it reaches high levels. Similarly, other chemicals like serotonin and norepinephrine help regulate sleep-wake cycles.

Physical Needs: Infants have physical needs that can disrupt sleep, such as hunger. Their small stomachs empty quickly, requiring frequent feedings both day and night. This need can often overlap or interfere with their sleep cycles.

While these biological and neurological factors provide a basic framework for understanding infant sleep, it is crucial to remember that they do not act in isolation. The external world and the environment in which an infant lives and grows play an equally crucial role. External stimuli, daily routines, and even the physical environment can have a significant impact on how and when an infant sleeps.

In section 2.2, we will explore these external influences in more depth, such as lighting, noise, and temperature, and how they can interact and influence the complex biological and neurological processes just described. The goal is to provide parents with a holistic view of infant sleep, helping them effectively navigate and manage both the internal and external aspects of their child's sleep.

2.2 External Environmental Influences

The external environment in which an infant lives and grows is a powerful and often underestimated force in regulating and shaping sleep. While internal biological and neurological factors play a role, external stimuli can either facilitate or hinder the establishment of a healthy sleep routine.

Light: As mentioned earlier, light influences melatonin production. Strong exposure to light, especially blue light emitted by electronic screens in the evening, can delay melatonin production, making the infant more active and less inclined to sleep. Conversely, exposure to natural light during the day can help synchronize the infant's circadian rhythm with the natural day-night cycle.

Noise: While some infants seem able to sleep through almost any type of sound distraction, loud or sudden noises can easily wake others. However, a background of white noise or soothing sounds, such as the sound of water or a gentle lullaby, can mask other environmental sounds and help the infant sleep more deeply.

Temperature and Comfort: A room temperature that is too hot or too cold can disturb sleep. Ideally, the room should be cool, but the infant should be adequately covered. The choice of sheets and clothing can also influence sleep quality: natural and breathable materials like cotton can offer greater comfort.

Parental Presence and Absence: The sense of security provided by the proximity of parents can influence an infant's sleep. Some families choose co-sleeping, while others opt for separate cribs. Regardless of the choice, consistency and safety are crucial. The infant should feel that, even if they don't see the parents, they are there for them.

Stimulation Before Bedtime: An overstimulating environment, with energetic play or excessive interaction before bedtime, can overly excite the *infant and make falling asleep more difficult. A quiet and relaxing routine, on the other hand, can signal to the baby's brain that it's time to calm down and prepare for sleep.*

By understanding and adapting to these environmental factors, parents can create an optimal sleep environment for their infants. However, it's crucial to remember that the external environment doesn't act alone; it interacts and intertwines with family routines and habits, representing another crucial aspect of sleep regulation.

In the next section, 2.3, we will delve into how family routines, from feeding habits to time management, influence and are influenced by infant sleep. We will also provide tips on establishing solid and consistent routines that promote healthy and restful sleep for the entire family.

2.3 Family Habits and Routines

Family habits and routines play a fundamental role in determining the quality and quantity of an infant's sleep. While the external environment has its influence, it is the family's daily choices and practices that have the most direct impact on the infant. Understanding this connection is essential to ensure healthy sleep for the little one.

Bedtime Routine: A consistent bedtime routine provides clear signals to the infant that it's time to sleep. This might include activities like reading a story, singing a lullaby, having a calm bath, or simple cuddling. The key is repetitiveness: when the child begins to recognize a sequence of events preceding sleep, they can mentally and physically prepare to rest.

Meal Timing: Digestion can impact sleep. Feeding the infant regularly and ensuring they are neither too hungry nor too full before sleep can help avoid nighttime awakenings. Consistency in meal timings can also assist in regulating the infant's internal clock.

Family Interactions: Infants are highly sensitive to the atmosphere at home. Tensions, arguments, or stress can negatively influence their sleep. Similarly, a loving, calm, and supportive environment can help them feel secure and relaxed, facilitating deeper sleep.

Quality Time Spent Outdoors: As mentioned in the section on the environment, natural light helps synchronize the internal clock. Spending time outdoors, perhaps on a quiet walk, can help establish a good sleep routine while providing mental and physical health benefits for both the child and parents.

Technology Use: Excessive use of electronic devices in the family routine can influence melatonin production, not only in infants but also in parents. Limiting the use of such devices in the evening hours and creating a "technology-

free" environment in the infant's room can be beneficial.

It's important to emphasize that there is no "one-size-fits-all" when it comes to family routines. Each family is unique, and what works for one may not work for another. The key is experimentation and observation: noticing how the infant responds to different routines and adapting accordingly. Family habits are just one piece of the puzzle. Sometimes, despite the best intentions and well-established routines, some health issues may intervene and disrupt the infant's sleep. In the next section, 2.4, we will delve into these common health issues that can affect sleep and discuss how to proactively address them to ensure peaceful nights for both the child and the family.

2.4 Common Health Issues Affecting Sleep

An infant's health is delicate, and sometimes, despite well-established routines, health issues can arise that affect sleep. Identifying and understanding these problems is crucial for addressing them correctly and ensuring peaceful sleep.

Gastroesophageal Reflux Disease (GERD): This is one of the most common causes of sleep disturbances in infants. GERD causes food to come back up from the lower esophageal sphincter, causing discomfort. It can be identified by symptoms such as crying after meals, frequent regurgitation, or irritability when lying down. Dietary changes or slight elevation of the head during sleep can help.

Colic: If an infant cries excessively, especially in the evening hours, they may be suffering from colic. It's not yet clear what exactly causes colic, but consulting a pediatrician and finding ways to comfort the infant, such as swaddling or gentle rocking, is essential.

Ear Infections: An ear infection can cause pain and discomfort, especially when the baby is lying horizontally. If an infant shows signs of irritability or begins pulling their ear, a medical visit may be necessary.

Teething: Teething can begin as early as a few months and can cause discomfort and sleep problems. Swollen gums, excessive drooling, and an increased need to bite can be signals. Chilled teething rings or gentle gum massages can provide relief.

Allergies or Food Intolerances: If an infant experiences stomach issues, excessive gas, or irregular bowel movements after eating, they may have a food intolerance or allergy. It's essential to consult a pediatrician if a food reaction is suspected.

In addition to physical problems, infants can be influenced by emotional factors, which may manifest through their sleep. It might be surprising, but even infants can experience forms of stress or anxiety related to their environment or changes in their daily routine. In these cases, they might show signs like restless sleep, uncontrollable crying, or frequent awakenings. The connection between physical and emotional issues is close, and sometimes it's a combination of both that disturbs the infant's sleep. For example, a physical issue like reflux can cause discomfort, which, in turn, can generate stress or anxiety in the infant, further exacerbating sleep disturbances.

In conclusion, it's crucial for parents to be aware and proactive in identifying any health problems that could affect their little ones' sleep. Regular communication with the pediatrician, along with careful observation of the child's signals, can help intervene promptly. In the next section, 2.5, we will explore in more detail how anxiety and other emotional issues can manifest in infants and how parents can support and comfort their little ones during these challenging times.

2.5 Anxiety and Other Emotional Issues in Infants

Many parents are surprised to learn that even infants can experience emotional issues such as anxiety or stress. Although their young brains are still developing, they are already sensitive to the surrounding environment and the emotions of the people around them.

Recognizing Signs of Anxiety:
While adults can express their feelings verbally, infants communicate through behavior. Signals like inconsolable crying, frequent awakenings, irritability, or a decrease in appetite may indicate that an infant is experiencing anxiety.

Causes of Anxiety in Infants:
Infants can pick up on tensions in the family environment. Arguments, raised voices, or parental stress can influence them. Changes in routine, such as introducing solid foods or starting daycare, can also cause anxiety.
The Parent-Infant Bond:

A secure and stable connection with a parent or primary caregiver is essential for the infant's emotional well-being. This bond serves as a kind of "anchor," helping the infant feel secure even when exposed to new experiences or challenges.

Methods to Calm an Anxious Infant:
Gently rocking the infant, singing a lullaby, or even just maintaining eye contact and speaking in a calm voice can help soothe an anxious child. Skin-to-skin contact is another effective technique; physical closeness helps the infant feel the parent's heartbeat and calms them.

When to Seek Help:
If an infant shows persistent signs of anxiety or stress, and comforting techniques don't seem to work, it might be time to consult a pediatrician or a specialist in infant mental health. These professionals can provide guidance and specific suggestions on helping the infant better manage their emotions.

It's important to emphasize that all infants are unique and react differently to stimuli and challenges. What might cause stress or anxiety in one infant may not have the same effect on another. However, the key lies in observing, listening, and responding to the infant's needs with love and patience.

At this point, having explored in detail how physical and emotional issues can influence infant sleep, in the next chapter, 3.1, we will focus on the interaction between feeding and sleep quality. We'll discover how certain foods or meal timings can impact, both positively and negatively, the sleep of the little ones. This section will be particularly useful for parents who are beginning to introduce solid foods into their child's diet or are looking for dietary solutions to improve their infant's nights.

3.1 The Relationship Between Feeding and Sleep Quality

The feeding of an infant plays a crucial role in the quality and duration of sleep. What an infant eats, and when they eat it, can directly influence their ability to sleep soundly at night. As we explore this connection, it is essential for parents to understand how to balance the nutritional needs of the infant with the desire to ensure they sleep well.

Feeding Timing:
The timing of an infant's feeding can influence their sleep. Feeding an infant just before putting them to bed can help them feel full and relaxed, promoting longer sleep. However, it is crucial to ensure that the baby burps properly to avoid discomfort during sleep.

Introduction of Solid Foods:
Many parents hope that introducing solid foods will improve the sleep quality of their infants. While some studies suggest that infants who

consume solid foods earlier might sleep more, it is essential to introduce new foods gradually and monitor the baby for any signs of allergies or intolerances.

Effects of Stimulating Foods:
Even though infants do not consume caffeine like adults, they can still be exposed to it through breast milk. Breastfeeding mothers should moderate caffeine intake to prevent the infant from becoming restless or having difficulty sleeping.

Nighttime Feeding:
During the first few months of life, it is normal for infants to wake up at night to feed. However, as they age, many infants begin to reduce nighttime feedings. Parents can gradually try to decrease nighttime feeding by encouraging the infant to consume more during the day and ensuring they receive enough calories.

Hydration Benefits:

Although the primary source of hydration for infants is milk, it is essential to monitor signs of dehydration, especially in warmer months. Proper hydration helps regulate the infant's body temperature and promotes deep sleep.

As we explore the relationship between feeding and sleep, it is important to remember that every child is unique. What works for one infant may not work for another. Parents should be prepared to experiment and adapt to their baby's needs, always under the guidance of a pediatrician.

With this information in mind, in the next section, 3.2, we will delve further into the importance of breastfeeding compared to formula feeding. We will discuss the nutritional, emotional, and sleep-related benefits of breastfeeding and how it compares to the use of formula. Since this is a delicate topic subject to various opinions, it is crucial to approach it with a balanced and informative perspective.

3.2 The Importance of Breastfeeding vs. Formula Feeding

The debate between breastfeeding and formula feeding is as old as the history of motherhood itself. Each option has its advantages and disadvantages, and the decision on which path to take often relies on personal, cultural, and health considerations. Exploring these two feeding methods will help us better understand how they can influence the infant's sleep and overall health.

Nutritional Benefits of Breastfeeding:
Breast milk is rich in essential nutrients for the infant's development. It contains a perfect mix of proteins, fats, vitamins, and antibodies that help protect the child from diseases. This unique composition also helps regulate the baby's digestive system, potentially reducing issues like colic and gas that can disrupt sleep.

Emotional Connection and Security:
Breastfeeding not only provides nourishment but also fosters a deep connection between mother and child. This emotional bond can have calming effects on the infant, facilitating the transition to a deeper and more restful sleep.

Formula Feeding and Convenience:
While breastfeeding has many advantages, formula feeding can offer greater flexibility. Parents can precisely measure the amount of milk the infant is consuming, making it easier to establish a feeding routine. Additionally, it allows other family members to participate in feeding, giving the mother breaks and enabling the partner or other caregivers to bond with the baby.

Components of Formula Milk:
Modern formula milks are designed to come as close as possible to the composition of breast milk. They contain vitamins, minerals, and other essential nutrients for the baby's growth and development. However, the lack of natural

antibodies may make formula-fed infants slightly more susceptible to infections and illnesses.

Influence on Sleep:
Some studies suggest that formula-fed infants might sleep longer at night. This could be due to the fact that formula is digested more slowly than breast milk. However, it is essential to note that every child is unique, and what works for one may not work for another.

The choice between breastfeeding and formula feeding is deeply personal and should be based on what works best for the family and the infant. Consulting a pediatrician or a lactation consultant can help parents make an informed decision.

With this overview of breastfeeding and formula feeding, in the next section, 3.3, we will focus on meal timing and frequency. Understanding when and how often to feed the infant can make a significant difference in establishing a healthy sleep routine and ensuring the baby is satisfied and content.

3.3 Meal Timing and Frequency

Every infant is a unique individual, and as such, their dietary needs can vary significantly from one child to another. However, there are general guidelines and strategies that parents can adopt to optimize meal timing and frequency, positively influencing their little one's sleep.

Meal Frequency in the Early Months:
In the first months of life, infants require frequent meals both day and night. Most newborns need to be fed every 2-3 hours, amounting to 8-12 meals per day. This frequency is due to their small stomach volume and the rapid digestion rate of breast milk. However, with the use of formula, which tends to be denser and less easily digestible, some infants may stay satisfied for longer, extending the interval between meals.

Recognizing Hunger Cues:
Rather than strictly adhering to a schedule, it is advisable for parents to learn to recognize their baby's hunger cues. These include moving hands towards the mouth, making sucking sounds, or seeking the breast or bottle. Crying is often a late sign of hunger; ideally, you'd want to begin feeding the baby before it reaches that point.

Routine is Key:
Despite the importance of responding to hunger cues, establishing a daytime feeding routine can help predict and plan meals. A routine also aids in avoiding overfeeding and ensures that the baby receives the necessary nutrition during the day, promoting a higher likelihood of uninterrupted sleep at night.

Introduction of Solid Foods:
Around 6 months, many infants start showing interest in solid foods. This is an exciting milestone but can also lead to changes in the sleep routine. As new foods are introduced, it is crucial to monitor the baby for any signs of

allergies or intolerances and take note of how these new foods may influence their sleep.

Adapting to Evolving Needs:
As the child grows, their dietary needs will change. They might begin to eat more during each meal and require less frequent meals. Being flexible and adapting to these evolving needs can ensure that the baby stays satisfied and well-nourished, promoting quality sleep.

With a clear understanding of meal timing and frequency, it is important to recognize that, at times, despite the best efforts of parents, the infant may experience digestive issues that affect their sleep. In the next section, 3.4, we will delve into these digestive issues and how they might interact with the infant's sleep routine, offering suggestions on managing and preventing these challenges.

3.4 Digestive Issues and Sleep Disturbances

Infants, with their digestive systems still in the developmental stage, can be particularly sensitive to various digestive issues. These disorders often have a direct impact on the quality and quantity of sleep. Understanding and addressing these problems can make a significant difference in the nightly serenity of an infant and, consequently, the entire family.

Colic:
One of the most common digestive issues in infants is colic. Characterized by intense and prolonged crying, often during the evening, colic can result from trapped gas or intestinal spasms. Although the exact cause of colic remains partly a mystery, we know that it can be extremely stressful for parents and can disrupt the baby's sleep.

Gastroesophageal Reflux (GERD):
Some infants may suffer from reflux, where small amounts of food come back up the esophagus,

causing discomfort or even pain. This can make the baby restless during sleep and lead to frequent awakenings. Elevating the baby's head slightly during sleep and ensuring they remain upright for a while after meals can help.

Food Intolerances and Allergies:
In some cases, an infant might react to certain foods or components of breast milk or formula. These reactions can range from mild to severe, manifesting through symptoms like rashes, diarrhea, vomiting, or sleep problems. If food intolerance or allergy is suspected, it is crucial to consult a pediatrician.

Constipation:
Though rare, constipation can occur in infants, especially with the introduction of solid foods. A constipated baby might sleep irregularly or appear particularly irritable. Ensuring the baby receives an adequate amount of liquids and discussing the introduction of fiber-rich foods with a doctor can help.

Gas and Bloating:
Air ingestion during breastfeeding or bottle-feeding, or reactions to certain foods, can cause gas and bloating. This can result in a restless, disturbed-sleeping baby. Techniques such as burping the baby after meals or using anti-colic bottles can be helpful.

The key to managing these digestive issues is prevention and careful observation. Parents should closely monitor their child's reactions to certain foods, and when something seems to cause discomfort, it's essential to discuss it with a healthcare professional.

However, it's not just about what might cause problems; there are also foods that can promote healthy digestion and potentially better sleep. In the next section, 3.5, we will explore foods that can be particularly beneficial for an infant's sleep, as well as those that might be best avoided, providing an overview of how nutrition can effectively promote restful nights.

3.5 Foods to Avoid and Those Recommended

The nutrition of an infant is a fundamental aspect that influences their growth, development, and sleep quality. While breast milk or formula is the primary source of nourishment in the early months of life, the introduction of solid foods is a crucial stage that can impact sleep. To help parents make informed choices, let's explore recommended and to-be-avoided foods.

Foods to Avoid:

Spicy or Highly Seasoned Foods:

While they may not directly cause digestive issues, they can irritate the infant's delicate system, leading to sleepless nights.
Some Dairy Products:

Some children may show sensitivity to dairy products, manifesting as gas, diarrhea, or

rashes. If intolerance is suspected, consulting the pediatrician is advisable.
Acidic Fruits:

Fruits like citrus or pineapples may cause acidity or rashes in some infants.
High Nitrate Foods:

Such as spinach or beets. These can be introduced later once the baby's digestive system has further developed.
Caffeine:

Present in chocolate or some sweets. It can stimulate the baby and disrupt their sleep.
Recommended Foods:

Whole Grains:

Such as brown rice or oats, can be easy to digest and provide a sustained energy release, promoting peaceful sleep.
Leafy Green Vegetables:

Provide iron and are rich in essential nutrients. They are easy to puree and introduce as one of the first solid foods.

Sweet Fruits like Pears or Apples:

These can be cooked and pureed, offering essential vitamins without the acidity of other fruits.

Lean Proteins like Chicken or Turkey:

They are a good source of protein and iron, and are generally easy to digest.

Legumes:

Such as lentils or chickpeas, can be gradually introduced and are a good source of protein and fiber.

While navigating the complex world of infant feeding, it is essential to observe how the child reacts to new foods. Every child is unique, and what works for one may not work for another. As the child grows and their digestive system matures, experimenting with a wider range of foods is possible, always paying attention to the child's signals. Now that we have explored how nutrition can influence sleep, in the next chapter, we will delve into the world of sounds, examining how certain noises can effectively promote deep and restful sleep. Section 4.1, "What Are White Noises and Why Do They Work," will unveil the mystery behind these sounds and why they have become a popular ally for parents in promoting peaceful sleep for their little ones.

4.1 What Are White Noises and Why Do They Work

In the heart of the night, when every little noise seems amplified, and each awakening of the baby can feel like an eternity, many parents have found an unexpected ally: white noise. But what exactly is meant by "white noise," and why does it seem to have such a soothing effect on infants?

Definition of White Noise:
White noise, in technical terms, is a signal that has constant intensity across all audible frequencies. Imagine it as a steady hum or hiss that sounds uniformly across the entire spectrum of hearing. To simplify, it's similar to the sound of a running fan, rainfall, or a radio tuned to a frequency without a station.

Biological Origins of White Noise Effectiveness:
The reason why white noise works so well with infants might have evolutionary roots. In the womb, babies are exposed to a range of

continuous sounds, such as the mother's heartbeat, blood flow, and other internal sounds. This sonic environment may resemble, in certain ways, white noise. Therefore, once born, white noises can remind infants of that familiar and reassuring context, providing a sense of security and comfort.

Masking Background Noises:
Another advantage of white noise is its ability to mask or drown out other sounds. Living in a noisy world with traffic sounds, conversations, TVs, and more, it can be challenging for a baby to sleep deeply without being disturbed. White noise creates a kind of "sound cushion" that can muffle or cover these disruptive noises.

Promoting Deeper and More Restful Sleep:
Studies have suggested that white noise can help not only with falling asleep but also with maintaining deep sleep. This can be particularly helpful during daytime naps when the environment might naturally be noisier.

Safety Considerations:

It is crucial to emphasize that while white noise can be helpful, it should be used safely. The volume should never be too high, and white noise sources should be placed at a safe distance from the baby's crib or bed. Constant exposure to high volumes can be harmful to the developing hearing of the child.

In conclusion, white noise has earned its reputation as a parent's ally in the quest for better sleep not by chance. It provides a sense of familiarity, masks disruptive sounds, and can promote deeper and more restful sleep. However, as with any tool, it is essential to use it appropriately and safely. In the next section, 4.2 "Useful Applications and Devices for White Noises," we will explore various options available for parents looking to incorporate white noise into their children's sleep routine, ensuring effective and safe use.

4.2 Useful Applications and Devices for White Noises

The effectiveness of white noise in facilitating peaceful sleep for infants has given rise to a wide range of dedicated applications and devices. These tools are specifically created to provide an optimal sound environment while ensuring ease of use and safety. In this chapter, we will explore some of the most popular options and how to select the one that best suits your baby's needs.

White Noise Machines:
White noise machines are standalone devices, often powered by batteries or a cable, that produce a range of sounds, including white noise, pink noise, and natural sounds like rain, waves, and wind. These machines often come with various settings, including timers, volume control, and sound selection.

Advantages:

Durable and designed specifically for use in nursery rooms.

Wide variety of sounds to choose from.

Some have additional features like night lights or projections.

Smartphone and Tablet Apps:

With the evolution of technology, it's not surprising that numerous apps are available that offer a wide range of white noise sounds. These apps can be downloaded onto mobile devices and often offer the flexibility to customize sounds.

Advantages:

Portable and always at hand.

Ability to combine sounds and create customized mixes.

Often updated with new sounds and features.

Plush Toys and Toys with White Noise:

For parents looking to combine comfort and functionality, there are teddy bears and other stuffed toys that emit white noise. These are often activated with a simple touch and can be cuddled by children.

Advantages:

Provide both tactile comfort and soothing sounds.

Easily portable.

Friendly and reassuring design for infants.

White Noise Audio and CDs:

Before the popularity of apps and dedicated machines, many parents relied on white noise audio CDs or files. These are still available and can be useful, especially if you have a CD player or another audio device in the baby's room.

Advantages:

Ability to loop for the entire night.

Various tracks to choose from.

How to Choose the Right Device:

Choosing the best device or application depends on individual needs. It's essential to consider portability, battery life, the variety of sounds offered, and any other features that might be important for the baby's sleep routine.

While using white noise can be a powerful ally in sleep, it's crucial to use it carefully. The next

4.3 Precautions and Duration of Use

The use of white noise can be a miraculous solution for many exhausted parents, offering that much-desired relief during sleepless nights. However, like any tool, there are precautions to take and guidelines to follow to ensure its use is safe and beneficial for the baby.

Hearing Protection:
The auditory system of infants is delicate and still developing. Exposing them to excessively high volumes can risk damaging their hearing. The golden rule is to keep the volume at the level of a soft conversation and place the sound source at a certain distance from the baby, not directly next to the crib.

Duration of Use:
While it might be tempting to leave white noise on all night, some experts suggest using it to help the baby fall asleep and then gradually decreasing the volume or turning it off altogether. This helps prevent potential

dependence on the sound to fall asleep in the future.

Sound Variability:
Even though white noise can be effective, it might be useful to vary the sounds from time to time. This can prevent excessive familiarity and adaptation, ensuring that the sound remains as effective as a sleep aid.

Recognizing Baby's Signals:
Not all babies will respond the same way to white noise. Some may find it reassuring, while others may appear agitated or disturbed. It's essential to observe the baby's reactions and adjust the approach accordingly.

Avoiding Dependency:
While white noise can be an excellent tool to facilitate sleep, parents should be cautious not to become overly dependent on it. The goal should be to help the baby develop healthy sleep habits, not to make them exclusively reliant on white noise to fall asleep.

Keeping the Room Safe:
When using electronic devices, such as white noise machines or cell phones, it's crucial to ensure they are placed in a safe position, out of the baby's reach and away from the crib, to avoid risks of suffocation or other hazards.

Considering Long-Term Use:
While the use of white noise can be particularly helpful in the early months of life, it may be worthwhile to assess whether to continue its use as the baby grows. Over time, the child may benefit from being introduced to other relaxing sounds, a perfect transition to our next topic, 4.4 "Other Relaxing Sounds for Infants."

In conclusion, while white noise has proven to offer numerous benefits in terms of infant sleep, it's essential to use it consciously and safely. The best approach is to balance the use of these sounds with other sleep techniques and always monitor and respond to the unique needs of your baby. In the next chapter, we will explore other sound options that can provide a relaxing environment and promote deep sleep for your little one.

4.4 Other Relaxing Sounds for Infants

While white noise has gained considerable attention as an effective means of calming and lulling infants to sleep, it's not the only sound that can have a beneficial effect. There are several other sounds, not classified as "white noise," that can provide a relaxing environment and facilitate deep sleep for your little one.

Nature Sounds:
Sounds like ocean waves crashing on the beach, birds chirping in the morning, or the sound of falling rain can have a calming effect on infants. These sounds mimic the uterine environment, where the baby was surrounded by various continuous noises, such as the mother's heartbeat and blood flow.

Heartbeat:
The sound of a heartbeat is one of the first and most familiar sounds a baby hears. Various products on the market reproduce the sound of a

heartbeat, offering the baby a familiar reassuring rhythm that can help them calm down and fall asleep.

Singing and Lullabies:
The human voice, especially that of parents, has an extraordinarily calming effect on infants. Singing a lullaby or simply speaking softly can provide comfort and security. The melody and rhythm of lullabies have the power to lull the baby into a drowsy state.

Classical Music:
Studies have shown that classical music, especially compositions by Johann Sebastian Bach and Wolfgang Amadeus Mozart, can have a positive effect on the developing brains of infants. Quiet and harmonious pieces can help soothe a restless baby and promote restful sleep.

Pink and Brown Noise:
In addition to white noise, there are other "colorations" of noise that can benefit infants. Pink noise, for example, has less energy in higher

frequencies, making it less sharp to the human ear. Brown noise, on the other hand, emphasizes low frequencies, resulting in a deep, rumbling sound.

Familiar Household Sounds:
The hum of a fan, the hum of an air conditioner, or the sound of a vacuum cleaner in operation can be reassuring for some babies. These constant and predictable sounds can provide a relaxing background that helps mask potentially disturbing noises.

Incorporating a variety of relaxing sounds into your baby's sleep routine can offer numerous benefits. Not only does it help the baby associate these sounds with bedtime, but it also provides a comfortable and familiar environment. However, as with white noise, it's essential to monitor the baby's reactions and make adjustments based on their individual needs. Having explored the wide range of relaxing sounds available, the next chapter, 4.5 "Integrating White Noises into Daily Routine," will discuss how to implement these *sounds into your baby's everyday life, ensuring a balance between sleep and wakefulness and providing the comfort of a familiar sound environment.*

4.5 Integrating White Noises into Daily Routine

As we've seen, white noise has the power to relax, soothe, and facilitate deep sleep for infants. But how can we effectively integrate this tool into a child's everyday life without it becoming a crutch or a disruptive element? Here are some guidelines and suggestions for implementing white noises into the daily routine.

Gradual Introduction:
As with any new element in a baby's life, it's crucial to introduce white noise gradually. Start with short sessions, gradually increasing the duration as the baby becomes accustomed.

Key Moments of the Day:
Identify specific times of the day when white noise might be particularly useful. These could include bedtime, naptime, fussy periods, or when there are external noises that might disturb the baby's sleep.
Consistency and Predictability:

Once white noise becomes part of the routine, it's important to keep it consistent. This regularity helps the baby recognize cues that it's time to relax or fall asleep.

Volume and Safety:
Ensure that the volume of the white noise is at a safe level. It should be slightly lower than the volume of normal conversation and never too close to the baby's ears. Hearing safety is essential.

Combination with Other Techniques:
White noise is just one tool at your disposal to help your baby relax. It can be combined with other techniques such as lullabies, gentle touches, or massages to enhance its calming effect.

Limit Dependence:
While white noise can be a powerful ally in sleep, it's crucial that the baby doesn't become overly dependent on it. Use white noise when

necessary, but try to vary techniques for calming the baby.

Different Environments:

White noise can be particularly useful when traveling or in an unfamiliar environment for the baby. It can provide a sense of familiarity and comfort even in new and potentially stressful settings.

Incorporating white noise into your baby's daily routine requires balance. While it can be a potent tool for facilitating sleep and calmness, like any other tool, it should be used wisely and mindfully. Always observe your baby's reactions, adjust based on their needs, and, above all, prioritize safety.

However, while the auditory environment in which a child sleeps is crucial, the physical environment also plays a fundamental role. In the next chapter, 5.1 "The Perfect Room: Temperature and Lighting," we will explore how to create the ideal sleep environment for your baby, considering factors such as temperature *and lighting. This will provide you with additional tools to ensure your baby has the best chances for healthy and restful sleep.*

5.1 The Perfect Room: Temperature and Lighting

The environment in which a child sleeps is crucial to ensure quality sleep. Environmental conditions such as temperature and lighting play a crucial role in creating a relaxing atmosphere conducive to sleep. Here's how to optimize these factors to ensure the best possible sleep experience for your baby.

Temperature:

Importance of Adequate Temperature:
The ideal temperature for a baby's bedroom should be between 18 and 20 degrees Celsius. This temperature range not only helps promote deep sleep but also prevents the risk of Sudden Infant Death Syndrome (SIDS).

How to Regulate Temperature:
If the room is too warm, consider using a fan or air conditioner. Conversely, if the room is too

cold, a thermostat-controlled heater or an electric blanket might be helpful. Always remember to keep these devices away from the crib for safety reasons.

Clothing and Blankets:
Depending on the room temperature, ensure the baby is dressed appropriately. Light cotton pajamas during warmer nights and heavier fabrics during colder nights. Blankets should be light and breathable, and the baby's face and head should remain uncovered to avoid the risk of suffocation.

Lighting:

Natural Light During the Day:
During the day, it's important to expose the baby to natural light. This helps regulate the circadian rhythm and establish a healthy sleep-wake cycle.

Soft Lighting at Night:
At night, it's crucial that lighting is soft. This helps the baby distinguish between day and

night. Using a nightlight or lamps with warm light can be helpful, especially during nighttime feedings or diaper changes.

Avoiding Blue Light:
Blue light, often emitted by electronic devices like phones, computers, and TVs, can interfere with melatonin production, the sleep hormone. To ensure optimal sleep, avoid exposing the baby to these lights at least one hour before bedtime.

Blackout Curtains:
Using blackout curtains can help regulate the amount of light entering the room, especially during the summer months when days are longer.

Creating the ideal sleep environment for your baby is a crucial step in ensuring quality rest. By carefully adjusting temperature and lighting, you can create a relaxing and comfortable atmosphere that promotes deep sleep. However, these are not the only factors to consider. In the next section, 5.2 "Choosing the Mattress and

Bedding," we will explore the importance of selecting the right materials to ensure safe and comfortable sleep. The right combination of environment, materials, and routine can make a difference in the quality of your baby's sleep.

5.2 Choosing the Mattress and Bedding

The baby's room has been set up considering ideal temperature and lighting. Now, let's turn our attention to another key element for the baby's sleep: where they will actually sleep. The choice of mattress and bedding plays a crucial role not only in the baby's comfort but also in their safety.

Mattress:

Firmness: It is essential to choose a firm and compact mattress for the baby. This prevents the risk of suffocation and provides suitable support for their growth.
Adaptability: While adult mattresses may have adaptive zones for various pressure points, for babies, a uniform mattress that does not conform excessively to their body is preferable.
Material: Some mattresses are made with natural materials, such as cotton or wool, while others are synthetic. It's important to check if the

mattress is free of harmful chemicals or potential allergens.

Waterproof Cover: A mattress with a waterproof cover is useful to prevent damage from accidents, such as milk leaks or diaper leaks.

Bedding:

Sheets: Opt for fitted sheets that fit perfectly on the mattress, without wrinkles or excess fabric. This not only ensures comfort but also reduces the risk of suffocation.

Breathable Materials: Cotton is an excellent choice for bedding as it is soft, breathable, and easy to wash. Muslin is also popular for babies due to its lightweight and breathability.

Avoid Padding and Pillows: For babies, it is advised to avoid pillows, quilts, and soft toys in the crib. They can pose a suffocation risk. Instead, you can use a lightweight and well-fitted blanket.

Theme and Design: While safety and comfort are of primary importance, the choice of bedding design and color can add a personal touch to the baby's room. However, it's crucial to ensure that all colors and designs used are non-toxic.

Maintenance and Cleaning:

Make sure to regularly wash the bedding to maintain a clean and hygienic environment for the baby. Use gentle detergents, and if possible, opt for fragrance-free products to avoid irritations or allergies.

A peaceful and rejuvenating sleep is influenced by the quality of the mattress and bedding chosen for the baby. Investing in quality, safe, and comfortable materials is a crucial step to ensure safe and pleasant sleep. Now that we have explored the importance of these choices, in the next section, 5.3 "Reducing Stimuli," we will focus on how a calm and distraction-free environment can further enhance the quality of your little one's sleep.

5.3 Reducing Stimuli

After selecting the ideal mattress and bedding, another fundamental aspect of creating a perfect sleep environment for the newborn is reducing stimuli. The surrounding environment, noises, lights, and even the air can influence the baby's sleep quality. That's why it's essential to minimize stimuli that can interrupt deep and restful sleep.

Noise:
Silent environments are best for sleeping, but it's not always possible to ensure absolute silence. Instead of trying to eliminate every single noise, it's better to create a constant background noise, such as that provided by white noise. This helps mask sudden or unexpected sounds that could wake the baby.

Light:
Newborns, like adults, sleep better in dark environments. Blackout curtains can be an effective solution to block external light. If a

night light is used, it should be dim and placed away from the crib. Blue light, in particular, can interfere with melatonin production, the sleep hormone, so choose lights with a warm hue.

Electronics:
Limit the use of electronic devices in the baby's room. Television, radio, or other devices can create visual or auditory stimuli that disturb sleep. Moreover, many electronic devices emit blue light, which, as mentioned, can interfere with sleep.

Movement:
Avoid sudden or abrupt movements in the baby's room while they are sleeping. Even if the baby might not wake up completely, unexpected movements can shift them from deep to lighter sleep, reducing the overall quality of their rest.

Air Quality:
Good ventilation is crucial. The room should neither be too dry nor too humid. A humidifier or dehumidifier can help maintain the right

balance. It's also important to ensure there are no sources of air pollution, such as cigarette smoke or strong fragrances.

Consistent Routine:
Maintaining a consistent bedtime routine can act as a signal for the baby's body, indicating that it's time to rest. This routine can include activities like reading a story, singing a lullaby, or giving a brief massage.

Reducing stimuli in the baby's room can make a significant difference in the quality and duration of their sleep. While some solutions can be easily implemented, such as using blackout curtains or eliminating electronic devices, others might require more attention and consistency, such as establishing an evening routine. However, while attention to reducing stimuli is crucial, it's equally vital to ensure that the sleep environment is safe. In the next section, 5.4 "Sleep Safety and SIDS Prevention", we will explore best practices to ensure that your baby not only sleeps deeply but also safely.

5.4 Sleep Safety and SIDS Prevention

In addition to ensuring a comfortable and stimulus-free sleep environment for your newborn, it is crucial to ensure that the sleep environment is safe. One of the biggest concerns for parents, especially in the early months of a baby's life, is Sudden Infant Death Syndrome (SIDS). This is a tragic condition where an apparently healthy newborn dies suddenly during sleep, and often the cause remains unknown. Fortunately, there are many precautions parents can take to reduce the risk of SIDS and ensure a safe sleep environment.

Sleep Position:
One of the most universally accepted recommendations is to place the newborn on their back to sleep. This position has shown to significantly reduce the risk of SIDS. Although the baby may turn on their own, it is crucial that, at least in the first few months of life, they are always placed to sleep on their back.

Clear Sleep Environment:

The baby's crib or cot should be free of unnecessary items such as plush toys, pillows, blankets, and padded bumpers. These objects can pose a suffocation risk. Instead, opt for a firm mattress and a fitted sheet.

Avoid Overheating:

As discussed in the section on the ideal room temperature, preventing the baby from overheating is essential. Dress the baby appropriately for the room's temperature and frequently check that they are not sweating or that their tummy is not too warm to the touch.

No Smoking:

Secondhand smoke is dangerous for newborns and can increase the risk of SIDS. Ensure that no one smokes in the house or near the baby.

Sleeping Close but Separate:

Sharing the room (but not the bed) with the newborn can reduce the risk of SIDS. This allows parents to easily monitor the baby and hear if any issues arise. However, avoid bed-sharing, as it can increase the risk of suffocation and entrapment.

Breastfeeding:
As discussed in the breastfeeding section, breastfeeding has many benefits, including the potential reduction of the risk of SIDS.

Use of Pacifier:
Some research suggests that giving the baby a pacifier during sleep may reduce the risk of SIDS. If you are breastfeeding, wait until breastfeeding is well-established before introducing the pacifier.

While SIDS remains one of the major concerns for parents of newborns, following these recommendations can go a long way in reducing the risk. Being informed and aware of best practices can help create a safe and serene sleep environment for your baby. However, ensuring sleep safety is only part of the equation. Creating a sleep routine, which we will explore in the next section, 5.5 "Creating a Sleep Routine," is equally vital to ensure that your newborn sleeps well and consistently. Consistency can work wonders for children's sleep and, consequently, the well-being of the entire family.

5.5 Creating a Sleep Routine

A routine is a fundamental pillar in a baby's life. Predictability not only helps the baby understand what to expect but can also provide parents with a sense of control in a period that can often feel chaotic. A well-structured sleep routine can facilitate quieter nights and more predictable daytime naps.

Importance of Consistency:
Consistency is key. Just as adults thrive on a daily routine, infants benefit from a predictable daily schedule. Going to bed and waking up at the same time every day can help stabilize the baby's internal clock, making it easier to fall asleep and wake up.

Bedtime Ritual:
A bedtime ritual is a series of relaxing activities that precede bedtime. This could include a warm bath, a lullaby, a short story, or gentle massages. These activities signal to the baby that it's time to wind down and prepare for sleep.

Familiar Environment:

As discussed in previous sections, the environment where the baby sleeps should be safe and comfortable. Keeping this environment consistent every night can reinforce the association between that place and bedtime.

Avoid Overstimulation:

In the hours leading up to bedtime, avoid overly energetic play or loud noises that might excite the baby. Soft lighting and quiet playtime can serve as an ideal prelude to sleep.

Monitor Sleepiness Cues:

Babies often give cues when they are ready to sleep. These may include rubbing their eyes, becoming irritable, or losing interest in the surrounding environment. Recognizing and promptly responding to these cues can prevent excessive tiredness, which might make it harder for the baby to fall asleep.

Be Flexible:
While consistency is crucial, it's also important to be flexible. If the baby doesn't seem tired at the usual bedtime or appears particularly sleepy earlier, adjustments may be necessary. Over time, you'll learn to recognize and adapt to your baby's unique rhythms.

While creating a sleep routine may require patience and experimentation, the long-term benefits are countless. A stable routine can promote healthy sleep, which, in turn, can positively impact the baby's development, mood, and overall well-being. However, beyond the routine, another fundamental aspect for healthy growth and secure attachment is physical contact.

Physical contact not only provides comfort and security to the baby but also has numerous health and developmental benefits. In the next chapter, 6.1 "The Importance of Physical Contact," we will explore the depth of this primal bond between parent and child and how it can positively influence sleep and the overall well-being of the newborn.

6.1 The Importance of Physical Contact

Physical contact is one of the most powerful tools parents have to communicate love, security, and comfort to their newborns. From the moment a child comes into the world, touch plays a crucial role in defining and strengthening the bond between parent and child, while simultaneously promoting the health and well-being of the baby.

Emotional Bond and Attachment:
The newborn's skin is extremely sensitive. Every caress, hug, or kiss is a reassurance of the love bond shared with the parents. These moments of physical contact help establish a strong attachment bond, crucial for the emotional and psychological development of the child. Secure attachment fosters greater trust, self-esteem, and the ability to cope with stress.

Physiological Benefits:
Various studies have shown that skin-to-skin contact, especially in the first hours and days of

life, has a profound impact on the health of the newborn. This type of contact can help stabilize the baby's body temperature, regulate heart rate and breathing, and increase oxytocin levels—an hormone associated with attachment and well-being.

Calm and Comfort:
Physical contact has a soothing effect on newborns. When a child is fussy or irritable, holding them or giving a gentle massage can calm them. The familiarity and warm presence of parents can work wonders in soothing a newborn.

Promotion of Growth:
Studies have shown that premature infants who receive regular touch and physical contact tend to grow faster and develop better than those who do not. Physical contact can stimulate the production of growth hormones in the newborn.

Aids Sleep:

Physical contact, especially skin-to-skin contact, can improve the quality and duration of a newborn's sleep. Many babies fall asleep more easily and sleep more deeply when cuddled or held close.

Physical contact is not just a way to reassure and comfort a newborn; it also has profound implications for their physical and emotional health. While modern society may sometimes emphasize the importance of independence and self-sufficiency from an early age, we must not forget the fundamental importance of physical contact in a baby's life.

This brings us to the next point, 6.2 "Newborn Massage Techniques." While spontaneous and casual contact is essential, there are also specific massage techniques that can further enhance the benefits of physical contact. These techniques not only strengthen the parent-child bond but can also help address specific issues, such as colic or sleep difficulties, while providing moments of relaxation and well-being for the baby.

6.2 Newborn Massage Techniques

Newborn massage has ancient roots and can be found in many cultures worldwide. It combines the power of physical contact with specific massage techniques to offer a range of benefits to both the newborn and the parents.

Benefits of Newborn Massage:
In addition to promoting a strong parent-child bond, newborn massage can help soothe a fussy baby, stimulate digestion, improve circulation, and even help a newborn sleep better. It can also provide relief from common issues like colic and constipation.

Preparing for the Massage:
Choose a time when the baby is relaxed but awake, ideally after a bath or before bedtime. Ensure the room is warm and draft-free. Use natural oils such as sweet almond or coconut oil, which are gentle on the baby's sensitive skin.

Basic Techniques:

Abdomen: With clockwise circular motions, gently massage the baby's abdomen. This can help release gas and alleviate constipation.

Legs and Feet: Take one leg in your hands and, with a gentle yet firm grip, glide down from the thigh to the foot. This helps relax the muscles. You can also gently massage the baby's feet by pressing lightly with your thumb.

Arms and Hands: Similar to the legs, glide down from the arm to the hand. Gently massage the baby's hands by opening and closing them softly.

Back: While the baby is lying on their stomach, make gentle "C" shaped movements along the entire back, avoiding the spine.

Face: Very gently, use the pads of your fingers to massage the baby's forehead, cheeks, and the area around the mouth.

Responding to the Baby:
During the massage, it is essential to observe and respond to the baby's signals. If the baby seems agitated or irritable, it might not be the right time, or they may not appreciate a particular movement.

Conclusion:
Conclude the massage with gentle, soothing movements, perhaps humming a lullaby. This leads to a natural transition to sleep or a moment of relaxation.

Newborn massage, therefore, not only provides physical benefits to the baby but also becomes a precious moment of connection between parent and child. And while touch is powerful in itself, voice also has surprising power, as we will explore in the next chapter, 6.3 "Singing and the Power of Lullabies." These ancient songs have calmed children for generations, offering comfort and security through melody and the familiar voice.

6.3 Singing and the Power of Lullabies

Music has always held a special place in human lives. From ancient Greece, where it was used for healing and soothing, to modern concert halls, it has continued to enchant generations. Yet, perhaps one of the most powerful and universal uses of music lies in the simple melodies parents have sung to their children for centuries: lullabies.

The Magic of Lullabies:
Lullabies are more than just songs; they are instruments of connection, comfort, and care. These melodies soothe not only through rhythm and melody but also through the familiar voice that sings them. The parent's voice becomes an anchor of safety, a signal that everything will be okay.

Benefits of Singing:
As the newborn listens to the lullaby, their heart rate may slow, breathing becomes more regular, and muscles relax. This response is not only due

to the melody but to the combination of sound, rhythm, and, most importantly, emotional closeness. Moreover, regularly singing to infants can enhance their listening and sound recognition skills, preparing them for language learning.

Voice as a Bonding Instrument:
Every parent has a unique voice, and for a newborn, that voice is a distinctive sign associated with comfort and security. When a parent hums or sings a lullaby, it's not just about the content of the song but the familiarity and consistency of the voice itself.

Choosing the Right Lullaby:
There is no universal lullaby that works for all children. Some may prefer gentle and slow melodies, while others might respond to more cheerful tones. The key is to experiment and observe how the baby reacts. Even if you're not a professional singer, what matters is the passion and emotion with which the song is presented.

Create Your Own Lullaby:
There's no need to stick to traditional lullabies. Parents can create their own melodies or adapt the lyrics of famous songs to make them personal. The essence of a lullaby lies in the intimacy and connection between parent and child, not in the perfection of the melody.

The Role of Lullabies in the Bedtime Routine:
Incorporating lullabies into the bedtime routine can help the child recognize that it's time to wind down and prepare for sleep. This daily ritual can act as a signal to the baby's nervous system, indicating that it's time to relax.

In conclusion, while techniques like newborn massage offer tangible benefits through touch, lullabies and singing play an equally crucial role in creating a relaxing and loving environment for the baby. And while the voice can calm and reassure, another effective way to prepare the baby for a peaceful sleep is through relaxing rituals, such as an evening bath, which we will explore in the next chapter, 6.4 "Relaxing Bath Before Bedtime".

6.4 Relaxing Bath Before Bedtime

The bedtime bath ritual isn't just a necessary moment for a baby's hygiene; it can transform into a profoundly relaxing experience and an effective prelude to sleep. Warm water, gentle hand movements caressing the skin, and a tranquil environment can synergize to prepare the baby for a night of rest.

Water as a Calming Element:
Water has an intrinsic power of relaxation. For a newborn, the aquatic environment can evoke the sense of security and protection from the mother's womb. A warm bath can help reduce tension and stress, also regulating the baby's body temperature in preparation for sleep.

Choosing the Right Products:
It's crucial to select gentle products specifically designed for a baby's sensitive skin. Opt for natural products without artificial fragrances or dyes that could irritate the skin or cause

allergies. Using essential oils, such as lavender, known for their relaxing properties, can further enhance the calming effect of the bath.

Massage Techniques in the Water:
The bath can be an ideal opportunity to introduce some massage techniques. Gentle circular movements on the baby's tummy, back, and legs can help them relax further. This practice promotes not only relaxation but also the bond between parent and child.

Create a Relaxing Atmosphere:
The choice of lighting and music plays a crucial role in making the bath a pleasant and relaxing experience. Soft lighting, perhaps achieved with a small night lamp, and a gentle background melody can create a serene and welcoming environment.

Establishing a Routine:
Like any other ritual, consistency is key. Choosing a fixed time for the bath helps the baby recognize and expect this moment of relaxation.

A well-defined routine can facilitate the transition from play and activity to calm and rest.

After the Bath:
Once the bath is complete, wrap the baby in a soft, warm towel, making them feel safe and protected. This moment can be used to cradle the baby, singing a lullaby or humming gently, further reinforcing the bond and emotional connection.

In conclusion, the evening bath is not just a hygienic gesture but a golden opportunity to promote the newborn's relaxation and prepare them for a night of deep and restful sleep. Integrated into a well-structured routine, which includes other pre-bedtime rituals, as discussed in the previous chapters, the bath becomes one of the pillars of preparing the baby for nighttime rest.
While the bath can be an excellent pre-bedtime practice, it's equally essential to establish subsequent rituals that gently guide the baby

into sleep. In the next chapter, 6.5 "Establishing Pre-Bedtime Rituals," we will explore strategies and techniques for creating a sequence of activities that lead to well-deserved rest.

6.5 Establishing Pre-Bedtime Rituals

Creating a solid and consistent pre-bedtime ritual is one of the most effective techniques to ensure that the newborn associates the moment of rest with specific relaxing activities. These rituals send clear signals to the baby's brain, indicating that it's time to slow down and prepare for sleep. Consistency and routine are crucial, and each family can create a ritual that best fits their needs.

Start with a Consistent Sequence:
Establish a sequence of activities that, once started, will lead to bedtime. It might begin with the relaxing bath we discussed, followed by a gentle massage, a story, or a lullaby. This sequence helps the newborn understand that once these activities commence, sleep will follow shortly.

Create the Right Environment:
Ensure the room is sleep-ready. Soft lighting, a comfortable temperature, and a gentle melody

or white noise can create an ideal atmosphere. Preparing the room this way every night can make the baby automatically associate that environment with rest.

Read a Story:
Even though newborns may not fully understand the words, listening to a reassuring parent's voice can have a calming effect. Choosing books with colorful and high-contrast images can also help gently stimulate the baby's vision.

Lullabies and Humming:
As explored in section 6.3, music and singing have a relaxing power. You don't need to be a professional singer; what matters is the melody and rhythm, combined with the reassuring tone of mom or dad's voice.

Offer a Comfort Object:
A soft plush toy or a blanket can become the transitional object the baby needs to feel secure. Ensure the chosen item is safe for infants, free of small or detachable parts.

Moment of Physical Contact:
Whether it's a brief cradle, a swing, or a hug, physical contact relaxes and reassures the newborn. This moment can be crucial for creating an emotional connection and strengthening the bond between parent and child.

Good Habits:
Avoid consuming foods or liquids too close to bedtime. Ensure the diaper is clean, and the baby is comfortable before putting them to bed.

Establishing pre-bedtime rituals not only helps create a relaxing environment for the baby but also provides parents with a special moment to share with their little one every day. These rituals, over time, become moments of growth and bonding that every family can treasure.

Continuing on our journey to ensure peaceful sleep for the newborn, we will encounter challenges such as colic, which can have a significant impact on rest. In the next chapter, 7.1 "Colic and Its Impact on Sleep," we will address this delicate topic and discuss solutions and strategies to manage these situations effectively.

7.1 Colic and Its Impact on Sleep

Colic poses one of the most significant challenges for new parents. These episodes of inconsolable crying, usually occurring in the first weeks of a newborn's life, can compromise the sleep quality of both the baby and the parents, leading to stress and anxiety. To address this issue adequately, it is crucial to understand the nature of colic and how it can affect the baby's sleep-wake cycle.

What is Colic?
Colic refers to episodes of intense and prolonged crying without an apparent cause. Babies with colic often cry at the same time every day, typically in the late afternoon or evening. The crying can last for a few hours, and despite the parents' efforts, consoling the baby may be challenging.

How Does Colic Affect Sleep?
Infants with colic often exhibit interrupted sleep. Episodes of crying may extend into the

nighttime, making it difficult for the baby to fall asleep. Additionally, the discomfort caused by colic can lead to frequent awakenings during the night.

What Causes Colic?
Despite abundant research, the exact cause of colic remains unknown. Some theories suggest it may be caused by gastrointestinal pain, the development of the nervous system, or even food sensitivities. However, none of these theories has been definitively confirmed.

Managing Colic and Improving Sleep:

Proper Nutrition:
If the baby is breastfed, the mother may consider monitoring her diet to exclude foods that can cause irritation. If the baby is formula-fed, discussing formula choices with a pediatrician may be helpful.

Upright Position After Meals:

Keeping the baby in an upright position after feeding can help reduce the risk of reflux and subsequent irritation.

Gentle Motion:

Rocking the baby or taking a short walk can provide relief. Consistent and rhythmic movement can have a calming effect.

White Noise and Music:

As discussed in previous chapters, soothing sounds can help relax the baby.

Skin-to-Skin Contact:

The closeness and warmth of the parent's body can provide comfort to the baby.

Consultation with a Professional:

If symptoms persist or are particularly intense, consulting with a pediatrician may be advisable to rule out other causes of discomfort.

Conclusion:

Colic can be a challenging and frustrating period for parents, but with patience, love, and the right strategies, it can be overcome. Although these challenges may impact sleep, establishing a solid sleep routine and adopting relaxing techniques can help navigate through these turbulent times.

While colic represents a temporary challenge, there are other aspects of infant sleep that parents should be aware of, such as sleep apnea. In the next chapter, 7.2 "Sleep Apnea," we will discuss these breathing pauses and how they can influence a baby's sleep.

7.2 Sleep Apnea in Infants

Sleep apnea, a condition characterized by temporary pauses in breathing during sleep, is a phenomenon that can cause concern among parents of newborns. Despite appearing alarming, it's important to recognize that not all forms of apnea are dangerous or abnormal in infants. In this chapter, we will explore what sleep apnea actually means for infants, its causes, and how it can be managed.

What is Sleep Apnea in Infants?
There are two main types of sleep apnea: central sleep apnea (CSA) and obstructive sleep apnea (OSA). In infants, central sleep apnea (CSA) is the most common. During an episode of CSA, the infant may stop breathing for a brief period, usually less than 20 seconds, due to a failure in the transmission of neural signals to the respiratory muscles. These episodes may be followed by a brief awakening or a movement, such as a small jerk.

Causes of Sleep Apnea in Infants:

Maturation of the Nervous System:
In premature infants, the central nervous system may not be fully developed, leading to episodes of CSA.

Infections:
Respiratory infections can cause episodes of apnea in infants.

Gastroesophageal Reflux:
In some cases, reflux can stimulate the vagus nerve and cause a brief pause in breathing.

Environment:
Factors such as an excessively warm room temperature can influence the frequency and severity of apnea episodes.

How to Manage and Monitor Sleep Apnea in Infants:

Monitoring:
Infants at risk, such as premature ones, may require continuous monitoring in the hospital to detect episodes of apnea.

Positioning:
Ensuring that the infant sleeps on their back can help reduce the risk of obstructive sleep apnea.

Avoiding Excessive Stimulation:
A calm and uninterrupted sleep environment can reduce the risk of apnea episodes.

Regular Check-ups with the Pediatrician:
Regular check-ups with the pediatrician are important to monitor the infant's growth and development and ensure that any episodes of apnea are not a cause for concern.

Conclusion:
While episodes of apnea can be concerning, in most cases, infants outgrow this phase as they mature and grow. It is always essential to consult a doctor or pediatrician to discuss any

concerns regarding the infant's sleep and ensure that all necessary precautions are taken. While sleep apnea is a specific aspect of infant sleep, there are other factors that can influence the infant's sleep-wake cycle. In the next chapter, 7.3 "Circadian Rhythm Disorders," we will delve into how the internal biological clock can affect the infant's sleep and how parents can help regulate this rhythm to ensure healthy and restful sleep.

7.3 Circadian Rhythm Disorders

The circadian rhythm, often referred to as the "biological clock," regulates the body's sleep-wake cycle and is based on the alternation between light and darkness over a 24-hour period. In newborns, this rhythm is not immediately established at birth, leading to periods of wakefulness during the night and sleep during the day. As they grow, infants begin to establish a more predictable circadian rhythm. However, there are times when this rhythm can be disrupted. In this section, we will explore circadian rhythm disorders in infants, their causes, and possible solutions.

Characteristics of Circadian Rhythms in Infants:
In the first few months of life, infants tend to sleep in blocks, regardless of whether it is day or night. This is entirely normal and physiological. However, around 3-6 months, many children begin to show a more defined sleep rhythm, sleeping for longer periods during the night.

Causes of Circadian Rhythm Disorders in Infants:

Light Exposure:
One of the main causes of circadian rhythm disorders in infants is exposure to light, especially blue light, during the evening hours. Devices such as mobile phones, tablets, and televisions emit blue light, which can interfere with the production of melatonin, the sleep hormone.

Feeding:
The timing and frequency of feeding can influence the infant's sleep-wake rhythm.

Activity:
Excessive stimulation or activity just before bedtime can disrupt the circadian rhythm.

Environment:
Environmental factors such as noise, temperature, and light levels can influence the circadian rhythm.

Solutions to Regulate the Circadian Rhythm:
Consistency in Routine:
Establishing a consistent sleep routine can help the infant recognize sleep-wake patterns.

Limiting Blue Light Exposure:
Avoiding the use of electronic devices in the evening and using soft lights or night lamps that do not emit blue light.

Proper Daylight Exposure:
During the day, it is beneficial for the infant to be exposed to natural light. This can help "reset" their biological clock and promote better sleep at night.

Create a Supportive Environment:
Ensure that the infant's room is quiet, dark, and at a comfortable temperature during the night.

Conclusion:
Regulating the circadian rhythm of the infant may take time and patience. However, with the right knowledge and attention to detail, it is

possible to establish a sleep routine that benefits both the infant and the parents.

As the infant's circadian rhythm becomes more predictable, other sleep-related issues with behavioral roots may emerge. In the next chapter, 7.4 "Behavioral Sleep Disorders," we will explore these challenges and discuss how they can be effectively managed.

7.4 Behavioral Sleep Disorders

Behavioral sleep disorders in infants and young children are common challenges that many parents face. Unlike disorders related to the circadian rhythm, these issues are often linked to specific behaviors or routines that can interfere with the infant's ability to fall asleep or maintain deep and restful sleep.

Types of Behavioral Sleep Disorders:

Sleep Onset Association Disorder:
Some children may become dependent on specific routines or objects (such as being rocked, sucking a pacifier) to fall asleep. If these conditions are not met, the child may have difficulty falling asleep.

Frequent Night Wakings:
While it is normal for infants to wake up at night, some may have difficulty falling back asleep without parental intervention.

Bedtime Resistance:
Some children may actively resist sleep, becoming hyperactive or irritable when it's time to go to bed.

Night Terrors:
Unlike nightmares, night terrors are episodes where the child wakes up in a state of panic but without a clear memory of a dream or nightmare.

Causes of Behavioral Sleep Disorders:

Inconsistent Routines:
Lack of a stable sleep routine can confuse the child's internal clock.

Excess Stimulation:
An overly stimulating environment before bedtime can make it harder for the child to relax.

Dependence on Specific Habits:
As mentioned, some habits can become sleep crutches.

Management Strategies and Solutions:

Establish a Consistent Sleep Routine:
Like circadian rhythm disorders, a stable routine can help signal to the child that it's time to sleep.

Create a Calm Sleep Environment:
Reducing stimulation before bedtime can help the child relax. This could include reading a story or listening to calming music.

Sleep Training:
Various sleep training techniques exist, some involving allowing the child to cry for increasingly longer periods before comforting.

Positivity and Reassurance:
It's essential for the child to feel secure in their sleep environment. Comforting the child after a night terror or nightmare can help reassure them.

Consult an Expert:
If sleep disturbances persist or become particularly severe, consulting a pediatric sleep therapist or pediatrician may be helpful.

Addressing behavioral sleep disorders can be a challenge for parents, but with the right understanding and strategies, these issues can be overcome. The key is consistency, patience, and attention to the individual needs of the child.

However, if, despite best efforts, sleep problems persist, or if there are other concerns about the child's health and well-being, it might be time to seek the advice of a professional. In the next chapter, 7.5 "When to Consult a Pediatrician," we will discuss signs and situations that might require specialized intervention.

7.5 When to Consult a Pediatrician

While every child has a unique sleep pattern and may go through phases where sleep is more disrupted, there are times when concerns about a child's sleep might warrant professional evaluation. Consulting a pediatrician or a pediatric sleep expert can provide reassurance to parents and, if necessary, action plans or targeted interventions.

Signs and situations that might require consultation:

Irregular breathing or breathing pauses:
If there are episodes where the child stops breathing for prolonged periods or has labored breathing, it is crucial to seek immediate medical attention.

Persistent difficulties falling asleep or staying asleep:

If the child regularly struggles to fall asleep or wakes up frequently without an apparent cause, discussing it with a pediatrician may be helpful.

Frequent night terrors:
While occasional night terrors can be normal, frequent or particularly intense episodes deserve attention.

Unusual sleep behaviors:
This includes rhythmic movements (such as headbanging against the crib), sleepwalking, or other atypical behaviors.

Loud or regular snoring:
Snoring may indicate issues like enlarged adenoids or obstructive sleep apnea in children.

Abrupt changes in sleep patterns:
If a child, who previously slept well, suddenly starts waking up frequently or has other significant changes in sleep, it could be a sign of health or developmental issues.

Benefits of consulting with a pediatrician:

Comprehensive assessment:
A doctor can examine the child to identify potential medical or developmental issues that might be affecting sleep.

Action plans and strategies:
An expert can provide practical advice and techniques to address specific sleep challenges.

Reassurance:
Knowing that one's child's sleep pattern is normal, or that there are solutions for any issues, can provide significant peace of mind to parents.

Referral to specialists:
If necessary, the pediatrician can refer to specialists such as pediatric sleep therapists, ear, nose, and throat specialists, or neurologists for further evaluations.

Conclusion:

The health and well-being of one's child are paramount. While many sleep-related issues may be temporary and part of normal development, it's always best to err on the side of caution and seek professional advice if there are concerns. Good sleep is fundamental for a child's growth and development, and by working together with the pediatrician, parents can ensure their child gets the rest they need.

Having addressed the crucial role of the doctor in evaluating sleep issues, in the next chapter, 8.1 "Understanding Night Wakings," we will focus on reasons why children might wake up at night and strategies for better managing and understanding these awakenings.

8.1 Understanding Night Wakings

Night wakings are a normal part of the sleep cycle for every individual, not just infants. However, for exhausted parents, each waking of their infant may feel like an unwelcome disruption. To better manage night wakings, it's crucial to understand the causes and nature of these awakenings.

Sleep cycles and night wakings:

Sleep is organized into cycles, including phases of light sleep, deep sleep, and REM (Rapid Eye Movement) sleep. During transitions between these phases, it's normal to experience brief awakenings. In infants, these sleep cycles are shorter than in adults, meaning they may wake up more frequently.

Common causes of night wakings:

Hunger:
In the early months of life, infants need to feed frequently, even during the night.

Discomfort:
This can include a wet diaper, a cold, or minor discomforts like reflux or teething.

Sleep habits:
If a child becomes accustomed to falling asleep only under certain conditions (e.g., being rocked), they might seek the same conditions when waking at night.

Overstimulation:
An overly stimulating environment before bedtime can make it challenging for the child to maintain deep and uninterrupted sleep.

Development and growth:
Periods of rapid growth or developmental "leaps" can temporarily disrupt sleep.

Managing night wakings:

While some night wakings are inevitable, there are strategies to manage them better and, in some cases, reduce them:

Calm and relaxing environment:
Ensure the child's room is dark and quiet. Using white noise, as discussed in previous chapters, can help create a relaxing auditory environment.

Recognize sleepiness cues:
Put the child to bed when they show signs of tiredness, such as rubbing their eyes or becoming irritable, to establish a more solid sleep routine.

Provide reassurance:
Sometimes, a brief touch or caress can reassure the child and help them go back to sleep.

Avoid the habit of feeding or rocking the child every time they wake:

If the child becomes accustomed to these conditions to fall back asleep, they might become dependent on them.

It's essential to remember that night wakings are part of normal child development. However, with a deep understanding of the causes and careful management, these moments can become more manageable for both parents and the child. The key is to strike a balance between responding to the child's needs and encouraging the development of healthy sleep habits.

In the next chapter, 8.2 "Self-Soothing Techniques," we will explore how to help children develop the ability to calm themselves and go back to sleep independently, a valuable skill that can contribute to reducing night wakings and ensuring quality sleep for both the child and parents.

8.2 Self-Soothing Techniques

One of the most crucial aspects of sleep in the early years of a child's life is the ability to self-soothe. This skill not only helps infants return to sleep after night wakings but is also a sign of emotional development and can positively impact their autonomy and security in the months and years to come.

What is self-soothing?

Self-soothing refers to a child's ability to calm themselves and return to sleep without external help from parents or caregivers. Some children may suck their thumb, while others may cuddle a stuffed animal or blanket. These behaviors are natural coping mechanisms that aid the child in relaxation.

Why is self-soothing important?

Besides allowing parents to have uninterrupted sleep, promoting self-soothing has several benefits:

Emotional development:
It helps the child manage stress and emotions.

Autonomy:
Strengthens the child's sense of independence.

Deep sleep:
Promotes quality sleep and more consistent sleep cycles.

How to encourage self-soothing:

Relaxing environment:
Ensure the child's room is a quiet and comfortable place. A familiar and calming environment can help the child feel secure when waking up during the night.

Comfort objects:
Providing the child with a soft stuffed animal or blanket can offer a sense of security. These items become positive associations with sleep.

Consistent routine:
A stable and predictable bedtime routine can signal to the child that it's time to sleep, helping establish a clear distinction between day and night.

Avoid immediate intervention:
If the child wakes up crying, instead of rushing to them immediately, wait a few minutes. This can give them the opportunity to self-settle.

Positive reinforcement:
If the child shows signs of self-soothing, praise them or acknowledge their efforts the next morning. This reinforces positive behavior.

Respecting the child's pace:

Every child is unique, and while some may learn to self-soothe relatively quickly, others might need more time. It's essential to respect the child's pace and offer support when needed.

While self-soothing is a desirable goal in managing infant sleep, it's crucial to remember that each child is an individual with specific needs and timelines. What works for one child may not work for another. Therefore, the key is to observe, listen, and adapt to the needs of your little one. In the next section, 8.3 "When to Intervene and When to Let the Child Be," we will delve into the delicate balance between supporting the child during night wakings and giving them the opportunity to learn to self-soothe independently.

8.3 When to Intervene and When to Let the Child Be

A newborn's sleep, especially in the first few months, is characterized by frequent awakenings. For parents, it can be a dilemma to determine when it's the right time to intervene and when it's more appropriate to let the child try to go back to sleep on their own. This decision requires balance, empathy, and an understanding of the child's individual needs.

Understanding the Signals:

Before deciding whether to intervene or not, it's essential to learn to recognize the child's signals. Not all awakenings are accompanied by crying; sometimes, a child might wake up, coo, or move for a few minutes and then go back to sleep. Intervening in these moments could paradoxically further disturb the child's sleep.

Different Types of Crying:

Crying is a means of communication for the newborn, and not all cries are the same. There's hunger crying, tiredness crying, or crying due to a wet diaper. Learning to distinguish between the different types of crying can help determine when and how to intervene.

The 5-10 Minute Rule:

A common practice suggests waiting 5-10 minutes when the child starts crying during the night. This interval gives the child the opportunity to self-soothe and return to sleep. If the crying persists or intensifies, it's time to intervene.

The Importance of the Environment:

As discussed in previous sections, a sleep-friendly environment can make a significant difference. Ensuring the room is at the right temperature, with relaxing sounds, and that the child is comfortable can reduce the need for nighttime interventions.

Sleep Training Methods:

Various methods exist to help the child sleep better and self-soothe, from "cry it out" to "gentle methods." It's crucial for parents to choose a method they feel comfortable with and that respects the child's needs.

Consistency is Key:

Whatever decision is made, consistency is crucial. If you decide to wait 10 minutes before intervening, it's essential to stick to this choice every night. This consistency will help the child understand what to expect and adjust their behavior accordingly.

Parental Sensitivity:

Lastly, every parent knows their child better than anyone else. If your instinct tells you something is wrong or your child needs you, listen to it. Your sensitivity and understanding of your child's needs are invaluable.

Whether choosing to intervene immediately or giving the child the opportunity to self-soothe, what truly matters is love, patience, and understanding. The sleep journey is an individual path for each family, and what works for one may not work for another. In the next section, 8.4 "The Importance of Partner Support," we will explore how teamwork and mutual understanding between parents can make a difference in managing infant sleep challenges and supporting each other during these demanding nights.

8.4 The Importance of Partner Support

The arrival of a newborn brings about a series of changes in a couple's life. Interrupted sleep, new responsibilities, and the constant need to care for a new human being can create tensions and unforeseen challenges. During this transitional period, mutual support between partners becomes crucial. Sharing responsibilities, communicating openly, and supporting each other can make the difference between a rewarding experience and a stress burden.

Clear and Open Communication:

The key to successfully navigating the challenges of the early months of a newborn's life is open and honest communication. Expressing emotions, fears, expectations, and needs can help prevent misunderstandings and unnecessary tensions.

Sharing Responsibilities:

Interrupted sleep can be one of the greatest challenges for new parents. Sharing the responsibilities of nighttime awakenings, such as establishing shifts, can help both partners get some rest and feel involved in caring for the baby.

Moments of Break:

It's essential to remember to take moments for oneself. This doesn't mean neglecting responsibilities but recognizing that to care for another human being best, one must first take care of oneself. This could involve enjoying a relaxing bath, reading a book, or taking a short walk—moments that can be supported and encouraged by the partner.

Empathy and Understanding:

Mutual understanding is crucial. One partner may feel more tired, stressed, or overwhelmed than the other at certain times. Recognizing and validating these feelings, rather than minimizing them, can strengthen the couple's bond.

Seeking External Support:

There's nothing wrong with seeking external support. This could include couples therapy, parenting support groups, or simply confiding in friends and family. Sometimes, an external perspective can offer valuable solutions and insights.

Remembering the Partnership:

It's easy to forget the couple's relationship when immersed in the responsibilities of parenthood. However, dedicating time to the couple, even through simple gestures like having dinner together or watching a movie, can help keep the bond alive and remind why they chose to become parents together.

Education and Training:

Informing oneself and getting trained on various parenting challenges, such as nighttime awakenings, can provide tools and strategies to better manage these situations. When both partners are informed, they can work better as a team.

Mutual support between partners during the first months of a newborn's life not only strengthens the couple's bond but also creates a loving and healthy environment for the baby. Remember that you are a team, and by working together, you can overcome any challenge that arises.

In the next section, 8.5 "Staying Calm During Night Awakenings," we will explore the importance of calmness and patience during nighttime awakenings and provide tips on how to best handle these moments.

8.5 Staying Calm During Night Awakenings

The night is silent, the world seems to have stopped, and suddenly, a sharp cry breaks that peace. It's a nighttime awakening. Every parent, especially in the first months of a child's life, has experienced this moment. And while it's natural for a newborn to wake up at night, the challenge for parents is to stay calm during these interruptions.

Understanding the Cause of the Awakening:

First and foremost, it's essential to understand that nighttime awakenings are a normal part of infant development. Children may wake up for various reasons: hunger, a wet diaper, need for comfort, teething, or even to assimilate new skills learned during the day. Understanding that there's nothing "wrong" can help manage the situation more calmly.

Deep Breathing and Counting:

In moments of stress or tiredness, a simple breathing technique can make a difference. Take a deep breath, hold for a few seconds, and then exhale slowly. Repeat a few times. This simple action can help calm the mind and prepare to face the child's awakening with more patience.

Avoid Checking the Clock:

One of the first actions many parents take when the child wakes up is to look at the clock. However, calculating how many hours of sleep have been lost or how much time is left until morning can increase anxiety. It's better to focus on the present moment and the immediate needs of the child.

Remember That It's Temporary:

Like every developmental stage, nighttime awakenings are temporary. Even though it might seem endless in that moment, children grow and change rapidly. This awareness can offer a reassuring perspective.

Create a Serene Environment:

Dim light, soothing music, or a gentle white noise can create a tranquil atmosphere that benefits both the parent and the child. A serene environment can facilitate the child's return to sleep and allow the parent to handle the awakening more calmly.

Avoid Comparisons:

Every child is an individual with their own rhythms and needs. Comparing one's child to others, or listening to stories from other parents about how their children "sleep through the night," can only generate stress and frustration. It's essential to remember that every family and situation is unique.

Staying calm during nighttime awakenings doesn't mean suppressing tiredness or emotions but rather facing these situations with understanding, empathy, and patience. The night may seem long, but with the right attitude and some strategies, it's possible to navigate through these moments with serenity and build an even stronger bond with the child. In the next chapter, we'll address a fundamental topic: recognizing parental stress in section 9.1. Understanding and addressing stress can significantly enhance the parenting experience and help establish a healthy and positive connection with the child.

9.1 Recognizing Parental Stress

Becoming a parent is one of the most profound and transformative experiences in a person's life. It brings immeasurable joys, moments of intimate connection, and the satisfaction of watching a new human being grow. However, along with these joys come challenges, responsibilities, and pressures that can lead to feelings of stress and anxiety. Recognizing and addressing parental stress is not only crucial for the well-being of the parents themselves but also directly impacts the development and health of the child.

Symptoms of Parental Stress:

The first step in addressing stress is recognizing its signs. These can vary from individual to individual but often include:

Feelings of constant fatigue or exhaustion, even after sleeping.
Irritability or brief outbursts of anger.

Difficulty concentrating or making decisions.
Feelings of isolation or loneliness.
Persistent anxiety or a sense of being overwhelmed.
Sadness or episodes of crying.
Changes in appetite or sleep patterns.
Reduced pleasure in activities that were once enjoyed.
Common Causes of Parental Stress:

While every parent may experience different sources of stress, some common causes include:

Lack of sleep or frequent sleep disruptions.
Social or cultural pressures to be a "perfect parent."
Conflicts or tensions with the partner regarding parenting.
Financial issues or concerns about the future.
Balancing work demands with family needs.
Worries about the child's health or development.
Feeling inadequate or unprepared for parenthood.
The Importance of Awareness:

Recognizing stress and admitting to feeling overwhelmed is not a sign of weakness. It is an act of awareness and strength. This awareness is the first step toward seeking solutions and adopting strategies to manage stress.

Talk About It:

Discussing one's feelings and concerns can be incredibly liberating. Whether sharing with a partner, a friend, a family member, or a professional, expressing emotions can provide relief and even bring new perspectives or suggestions on how to address challenges.

Don't Be Afraid to Seek Help:

There is nothing wrong with asking for help. It could involve asking a family member to care for the child for a few hours, consulting with a therapist, or participating in parent support groups.

Parental stress is a reality for many families, but recognizing and proactively addressing it can make a difference in ensuring healthy and balanced parenting. While taking care of one's well-being is crucial, it is equally essential to consider how parental stress can impact a child's sleep and development, a topic we will explore in the next section, 9.2. The emotional health of parents has a direct impact on the well-being of their children, making it essential to address and mitigate stress for the benefit of the entire family.

9.2 Impact of Parental Stress on Infant Sleep

Being a parent is one of the most rewarding experiences, but it can also be one of the most stressful. While much attention is given to the well-being of the child, we often overlook how the emotional state of parents can directly influence the sleep and overall well-being of the infant.

Emotional Connection and Sleep:

Newborns are highly sensitive to their surrounding environment and the emotions of those caring for them. An anxious, stressed, or tense mother or father may inadvertently transmit these emotions to the baby. This transmission can manifest in various ways, including sleep disruptions, difficulty falling asleep, or frequent awakenings.

The Role of Hormones:

When we are stressed, our bodies produce a hormone called cortisol. Although cortisol has vital functions, excessive levels can cause issues. During breastfeeding or simple physical proximity, there can be a transmission of these elevated cortisol levels to the baby, indirectly influencing their hormonal system and, consequently, their sleep patterns.

Awareness and Routine:

Children, especially infants, thrive on routine. A stressed parent may struggle to establish and maintain consistent routines, which can confuse the newborn and make it harder for them to establish a regular sleep cycle.

The Importance of Emotional Security:

A calm, loving, and stress-free environment provides the infant with a sense of security. This security is crucial for their emotional and physical development. When parents are stressed or anxious, they may inadvertently create an environment of insecurity, influencing not only the child's sleep but also their overall development.

Reaction to External Stimuli:

A stressed parent might overreact to minor disturbances or noises, waking the baby or making it harder for them to go back to sleep. This type of reaction can condition the baby to become more sensitive to external disturbances, further disrupting their sleep.

The Importance of Communication with the Partner:

Sharing concerns and stress with a partner or family member can help reduce the emotional burden. Mutual understanding and support are crucial for creating a serene environment conducive to the baby's sleep.

It is evident that parental stress has a direct impact on infant sleep. However, awareness of this connection is the first step to mitigate these effects. While trying to completely eliminate stress may not be realistic, there are techniques and methods that can help parents manage and reduce stress. Not only for their well-being but also to ensure that their baby has a calm and secure environment to grow and sleep. In the next section, 9.3, we will explore some relaxation techniques specifically for parents to help them navigate the challenges of parenthood without compromising the sleep and well-being of their child.

9.3 Relaxation Techniques for Parents

Being parents of a newborn can be incredibly stressful. From attending to the immediate needs of the baby to dealing with sleep deprivation, parents can feel overwhelmed. Therefore, having relaxation techniques at hand can significantly help reduce stress, improve sleep quality, and promote a more harmonious environment at home.

Deep Breathing:

One of the simplest yet most effective relaxation techniques is deep breathing. Inhale slowly through the nose, filling your lungs completely, and then exhale slowly through the mouth. This type of breathing helps calm the nervous system, reduce anxiety, and bring an immediate sense of calm.

Meditation and Mindfulness:

Meditation may seem like a complex art, but even a few minutes a day can make a big difference. Mindfulness meditation, in particular, teaches focusing on the present moment. Numerous apps and online resources guide parents through short sessions, ideal for those with limited time.

Stretching Exercises:

Physical and mental stress can lead to muscle tension. Spending a few minutes each day on stretching exercises can help relax muscles and promote a sense of well-being. The idea is not only to work on flexibility but also to connect with your body and release accumulated tension.

Warm Bath:

Immersing oneself in a warm bath, perhaps with the addition of bath salts or essential oils, can work wonders for the body and mind. It not only relaxes the muscles but also provides a moment of pause and reflection away from the demands of parenthood.

Music and Relaxing Sounds:

Listening to calming music or nature sounds can help soothe the mind. Put on headphones and let yourself be carried away by the sounds of ocean waves, gentle rain, or the melody of a piano piece.

Yoga Practice:

Yoga not only improves flexibility and strength but is also a powerful relaxation tool. Even a short 10-minute sequence can help restore inner balance and better manage stress.

Journaling:

Writing down emotions and thoughts can offer a form of release. Putting worries on paper helps put things into perspective and frees the mind from incessant thoughts.

Outdoor Time:

A short walk in the park or, if possible, in nature can work wonders. Fresh air, natural sounds, and movement help rejuvenate the mind and body.

Relaxation techniques are not just a way to escape the chaos of parenthood but a way to recharge and regain one's energy. When parents are relaxed and centered, they can offer the best version of themselves to their children. As we will explore in the next section, 9.4, a relaxed parent is also a parent who sleeps better. We will delve into the importance of sleep for both mom and dad and how good sleep quality can directly impact the well-being of the newborn.

9.4 The Importance of Sleep for Mom and Dad

While much attention is given to the baby's sleep, the sleep of parents is equally crucial. Becoming parents brings about a significant change in daily life and, as we've seen in previous sections, can be a source of stress and anxiety. Sleep becomes an even more fundamental element for the physical and psychological well-being of parents.

Physical Benefits of Sleep:

Sleep is not just a time for the body to rest; it is essential for a range of vital functions. During sleep, the body works to repair muscle tissues, renew cells, and strengthen the immune system. Sleep deprivation can lead to health issues such as weight gain, decreased immune function, and an increased risk of chronic diseases.

Sleep and Mental Health:

Adequate sleep is crucial for mental health. Lack of sleep can cause irritability, depressed mood, anxiety, and difficulty concentrating. For parents, this can translate to increased frustration, low patience, and a feeling of being overwhelmed.

The Domino Effect of Sleep Deprivation:

When one parent is tired, the other often feels the impact, creating a domino effect. A sleepless night can lead to tensions the next day, influencing communication and interaction with the partner and, in turn, with the baby.

Emotional Resilience:

Getting good sleep can help develop greater emotional resilience. With sufficient rest, it is easier to face daily challenges, stay calm in crises, and effectively manage stressful situations.

The Connection Between Sleep and Productivity:

Although it might seem counterintuitive, sleeping more can actually increase productivity. With a rested mind, parents can be more efficient in daily activities, better manage routines, and more easily find solutions to everyday challenges.

Sleep and Safety:

Sleep deprivation can lead to decreased reactivity and attention. This can be particularly dangerous when caring for a newborn. For instance, fatigue may make it difficult to hold the baby safely or react promptly to unexpected situations.

The importance of sleep for mom and dad cannot be overstated. While nighttime wake-ups and the demands of the newborn can make uninterrupted sleep challenging, it is essential to find ways to ensure that both parents get the rest they need. This might involve taking turns for nighttime feedings, taking restful afternoons when possible, or seeking help from family and friends to get some relief. Having deeply understood the importance of sleep for parents, in the next section, 9.5, we will explore how to find balance and support on this journey. As the saying goes, it takes a village to raise a child, and balance and support are the keys to successfully navigating this village.

9.5 Finding Balance and Support

When it comes to raising a newborn, balance and support are two keywords echoing continuously in every parent's experience. If the previous section emphasized the importance of sleep, now we explore how to manage responsibilities and seek support to maintain good mental and physical health.

Recognize the Importance of Balance:

The first step in finding balance is acknowledging its importance. Being a parent is one of the most beautiful yet demanding experiences. It's crucial to understand that to take the best care of your child, you also need to take care of yourself. This might mean taking a break when feeling overly stressed or delegating some responsibilities to other family members.

Schedule "Me" Time:

It's essential to schedule moments of pause and relaxation. Whether it's a short outdoor walk, reading a book, or practicing yoga, every parent should find an activity that allows them to disconnect and recharge. These moments not only help reduce stress but also make it easier to face daily challenges.

Ask for Help When Needed:

Many cultures emphasize the importance of community in a child's upbringing. Asking for help is not a sign of weakness but rather of strength. Whether it's grandparents, friends, or professionals, having a solid support network can make a significant difference in a parent's life.

Parental Support Groups:

Joining forces with other parents can be very beneficial. Participating in support groups, both online and offline, can provide a safe space to share experiences, challenges, and successes. Feeling understood and knowing you're not alone can help overcome difficult times.

Set Priorities:

Not everything that seems urgent truly is. Learning to set priorities can help parents manage their time and energy better. Some tasks can be postponed or delegated, while others, like quality time with the child or partner, should always be at the top of the list.

Communicate with Your Partner:

Open and honest communication with your partner is crucial. Sharing concerns, needs, and feelings can help both feel more supported and understood. This, in turn, strengthens the relationship and provides a solid foundation to build a family upon.

Finding balance and support is not always easy but is essential for the health and well-being of parents and, consequently, the child. As the saying goes, "You can't pour from an empty cup." Taking care of oneself, seeking support, and maintaining a balance between various responsibilities allow parents to offer the best to their children. After exploring the dynamics, challenges, and solutions for effective care of both newborns and parents, in the next section, 10.1, we will summarize the key strategies we've discussed. This will serve as a practical guide to navigate sleepless nights and challenging days with increased confidence and serenity.

10.1 Summary of Key Strategies

The journey through caring for newborns and adapting to life as new parents can feel like a rollercoaster of emotions, challenges, and unforgettable moments. Throughout this book, we've explored a variety of topics and solutions to help parents navigate these sometimes turbulent waters. In this chapter, we'll summarize the key strategies to ensure you have essential information at your fingertips.

Establish Bedtime Rituals:

Newborns respond well to routine. Establishing bedtime rituals such as a relaxing bath or reading a story helps the baby recognize that it's time to sleep, easing the transition into slumber.

Understand Sleep-Related Disorders:

From colic to night apnea, being informed about possible sleep-related disorders can help identify any issues promptly and seek a solution or medical help if necessary.

Self-Soothing Techniques:

Teaching the baby to self-soothe is not only a valuable skill for them but also provides parents with moments of respite. However, this must be balanced with knowing when to intervene.

The Importance of Mutual Support Between Partners:

Caring for a newborn is a team effort. Open communication, shared responsibilities, and mutual support are crucial for mental health and the well-being of the relationship.

Manage Parental Stress:

Recognizing signs of stress and taking preventive measures, such as relaxation and meditation, can help parents stay centered and present in daily challenges.

Prioritize Parents' Sleep:

While the focus is often on the baby's sleep, parents' sleep is equally crucial. Finding ways to rest, even if fragmented, can make a significant difference in overall well-being and the ability to face challenges.

Find Balance and Seek Support:

Every parent needs a support network, whether composed of family, friends, or support groups. These networks can offer practical help, advice, or simply a listening ear.

Conclusion of the Summary:

These key strategies, while not exhaustive, provide a solid foundation to assist parents on their journey. However, one thing to always keep in mind is the importance of flexibility. Despite preparation, every child is unique, and what works for one may not work for another. That's why the next section, 10.2, will focus on the importance of flexibility and adaptation, allowing parents to successfully navigate the unpredictable waters of parenthood.

10.2 The Importance of Flexibility and Adaptability

In the intricate universe of parenthood, if there's one universal truth, it's this: every child is unique. Despite the abundance of guides, advice, and strategies, what works for one child may not have the same effect on another. And this is precisely where flexibility and adaptability come into play, two key components in every parent's toolbox.

Flexibility: a skill, not a weakness.

Many times, society tends to view flexibility as a sign of indecision or lack of firmness. But in parenthood, flexibility is synonymous with strength. It means being intuitive enough to recognize when a strategy isn't working and courageous enough to change course. Rather than rigidly adhering to a predetermined plan, flexible parents are ready to modulate their approach based on the ever-evolving needs of their child.

Adaptability is key to growth.

As the child grows and evolves, so do their needs. What works in the early months may not be effective six months later. That's why, in addition to short-term flexibility, parents must also have the ability to adapt in the long term. This may involve updating routines, learning new techniques, or simply recognizing and accepting changes in their child's behavior.

How to cultivate flexibility and adaptability:

Self-reflection:

Take a moment now and then to reflect on what's working and what isn't. Self-reflection can help you identify areas where you might need to be more flexible or adapt to new circumstances.

Openness to change:

Embrace change as a natural part of the parenting journey. Instead of resisting, try to see each change as an opportunity to grow and learn together with your child.

Communication:

Communicate openly with your partner, family, or friends about how you feel and any challenges you're facing. Communication can offer new perspectives and solutions you may not have considered.

Continuous education:

The world of parenthood is continually evolving. Attend workshops, read books, or join support groups to stay updated and open to new techniques and approaches.

Acceptance:

Sometimes, things don't go as planned, and that's okay. Accept that perfection doesn't exist in parenthood, and every mistake or change of course is an opportunity for growth.

In conclusion, while strategies and techniques are valuable tools, the ability to be flexible and adapt to your child's changing needs is crucial. This dynamic approach will not only enhance your experience as a parent but will also help your child feel understood and supported. And as you navigate through these periods of change and adaptation, it's essential to remember that, like sleep, the relationship with your child will grow and evolve with age. In the next section, 10.3, we will explore how this relationship and sleep habits change as the child grows, offering a detailed insight into the evolution of sleep with age.

10.3 Growing Together: The Evolution of Sleep with Age

Sleep, like every aspect of a child's growth and development, is not static; it changes and adapts as the child grows. Understanding these evolutions can help parents navigate the changes with greater awareness and provide appropriate support at each stage.

Newborns (0-3 months): In this stage, newborns sleep a lot but wake frequently to feed. They don't yet have a well-defined circadian rhythm, meaning the difference between day and night may not be clear to them. The key in this stage is patience and creating a stable sleep environment with white noise, dim lights, and reassuring routines.

Infants (3-12 months): As infants grow, they begin to sleep more at night and less during the day. However, night awakenings can still occur, often due to developmental milestones or teething. A consistent bedtime routine, with calming activities such as a bath or reading, can help establish healthy sleep habits.

Toddlers (1-3 years): At this age, many toddlers have given up morning naps and take only one afternoon nap. Toddlers are known for their "escape" feats from the crib and "stalling" tactics at bedtime. The key is consistency: setting clear limits and staying firm can prevent many sleep-related challenges.

Preschoolers (3-5 years): While the need for daytime naps decreases, preschoolers may start experiencing nightmares or a fear of the dark. Reassuring them and creating a safe sleep environment is crucial. A small night light or a favorite stuffed animal can work wonders.

School-age Children (6-12 years): With the start of school and extracurricular activities, maintaining a regular sleep routine can become challenging. However, adequate sleep is crucial for learning and growth. Parents should monitor electronic device use before bedtime, ensuring children have a "quiet" hour before sleep to help them unwind.

Adolescents (13-18 years): Adolescent hormones can shift the biological clock, causing teenagers to stay up late and want to sleep in. Although they may seem independent, teenagers still need guidelines to ensure they get the rest they need. The key is dialogue and understanding.

As the child grows, it's essential for parents to grow with them, adjusting their strategies and expectations to the changing sleep needs of their child. Each stage presents its challenges but also its joys. And in every stage, support, understanding, and communication remain essential.

In the next section, 10.4, we'll have the opportunity to explore success stories and testimonials from parents who have navigated through these stages, offering a practical and reassuring insight into how they handled and overcame sleep-related challenges.

10.4 Success Stories and Testimonials

Personal stories have the power to inspire, reassure, and offer a real perspective on challenges and successes. Here are some testimonials from parents who faced and overcame difficulties related to their children's sleep.

Sara and Matteo: The Bedtime Ritual
"When Sofia was around 18 months old, she consistently refused to go to bed. After reading various books and consulting specialists, we introduced a bedtime ritual. Every evening, after dinner, we would read a story, sing a lullaby, and then tuck her into bed with her favorite stuffed animal. After a few weeks, she began to expect and love this ritual, and she stopped resisting bedtime."

Roberto and Chiara: Managing Nightmares
"At around 4 years old, Luca began having nightmares. Every night he would come to us,

terrified. Instead of sending him straight back to bed, we started talking about his dreams, giving names to the monsters and inventing stories where he was the hero defeating these creatures. This 'narrative therapy' helped Luca overcome his fears and sleep better."

Elena, Single Mother: The Strategic Nap
"As a single mother, sleep was a precious commodity. My little Lorenzo often woke up at night. I started noticing that he easily fell asleep during car rides. So, every afternoon, we would take a short drive, and he would nap. This afternoon nap worked wonders for his nights and made my life much more manageable."

Valentina and Marco: The Importance of Consistency
"With two twins, chaos was inevitable. But we realized that consistency was the key. Even when we were tired, we tried to maintain the same routine every night. This predictability helped our boys understand what to expect and made bedtime much less stressful for all of us."

Federico and Laura: Addressing Sleep Development Delays
"Our Tommaso had sleep issues well beyond infancy. After consulting a sleep expert, we discovered he had a delay in circadian rhythm development. With the help of targeted therapies and a lot of patience, we were able to regulate his sleep. This experience taught us the importance of seeking help when needed and being patient and loving, no matter the challenges."

These stories are a reminder that every family and every child is unique. There is no one-size-fits-all solution to sleep problems, but with love, patience, and sometimes the help of experts, solutions can be found.

In our next section, 10.5, we will explore how these challenges, though sometimes overwhelming, can actually strengthen parents' resilience and teach the importance of patience—skills that are invaluable in raising a healthy and happy child.

10.5 Encouraging Resilience and Patience

The journey of parenthood is filled with unexpected challenges, and among them, children's sleep issues often take a prominent place. However, like many difficulties we encounter in life, these challenges can become opportunities—precious moments to develop and strengthen qualities such as resilience and patience.

Resilience: The Art of Adapting and Overcoming

Resilience is not merely the ability to withstand adversity but rather the ability to adapt, learn, and grow through it. When we face sleepless nights, colic, night terrors, or any other sleep-related challenge, we are not merely "surviving" these moments; we are developing an inner resilience that will assist us in many other life situations.

For many families, overcoming these tough nights can become a symbol of what they can endure. The strength they discover within themselves during these challenging times makes them more prepared to handle other challenges life may present.

Patience: The Gift of Time and Love

Patience, like resilience, is a virtue that develops with practice. While it can be frustrating to soothe a restless child or wake up multiple times during the night, these moments also offer a unique opportunity to practice patience. Over time, we learn that each phase has its challenges but is temporary. And with this awareness, we can approach each challenge with a more peaceful and patient perspective.

Patience also teaches us the importance of time and love. Spending time with our children, even in the most challenging moments, strengthens our bond with them. And through this connection, we often find the strength and determination to persevere, even when things seem impossible.

The Legacy of Resilience and Patience

The lessons we learn as we navigate through sleep challenges benefit not only us as parents but also our children. Through our example, we show them how to face difficulties with grace, determination, and love. They grow up observing our resilience and learning the importance of patience. And, in many ways, what we teach them during these formative years prepares them for the challenges they will face in their lives.

As we close this chapter on parenthood and sleep, it is essential to remember that, although challenges may seem enormous at a given moment, they also offer invaluable opportunities for growth and development, both for parents and children. Through resilience and patience, we can transform these challenges into moments of learning and connection. And, in the end, these are often the moments we remember and cherish the most in our journey as parents.

Dear parents,

First and foremost, we want to tell you something fundamental: you are doing an extraordinary job. Being parents is a journey filled with challenges and joys, uncertainties and triumphs. In every moment, every day, you dedicate your love and dedication to the well-being and happiness of your child. This, in itself, is the greatest testament to your incredible work.

It's normal to face doubts, the fear of making mistakes, or not feeling up to the task. However, remember that there is no perfection in parenting. Every family, every child, every parent is unique. What truly matters is the love, patience, and commitment you put into raising your child.

The fact that you are seeking answers, trying to better understand the needs of your child, is the clearest evidence of your dedication. You are willing to learn, to grow, to evolve alongside your child. This makes parents true superheroes. Keep doing what you're doing. Let yourselves be guided by your love, your instinct, and never forget to take care of yourselves. You are your child's safe harbor, and to be that, you must also be your own safe harbor.

Be kind to yourselves, be patient with yourselves. Celebrate victories, learn from obstacles. And remember, you are not alone. We are here, your friends, your family, and an entire community of parents who share your experiences.

You are doing a fantastic job, and we are honored to walk alongside you in this wonderful journey that is parenthood.

If you think you liked and found this book helpful, I only ask you to take a few seconds to leave a brief review on Amazon!

Thank you,

Anna Silvestri